EMOTIONAL DETOX THROUGH BODYWORK

A Woman's Guide to Healing and Awakening

Mal Weeraratne

authorHOUSE®

AuthorHouse™ UK
1663 Liberty Drive
Bloomington, IN 47403 USA
www.authorhouse.co.uk
Phone: 0800.197.4150

Published by AuthorHouse 08/03/2018

ISBN: 978-1-5049-9415-6 (sc)
ISBN: 978-1-5049-9416-3 (hc)
ISBN: 978-1-5049-9417-0 (e)

Contents

Foreword

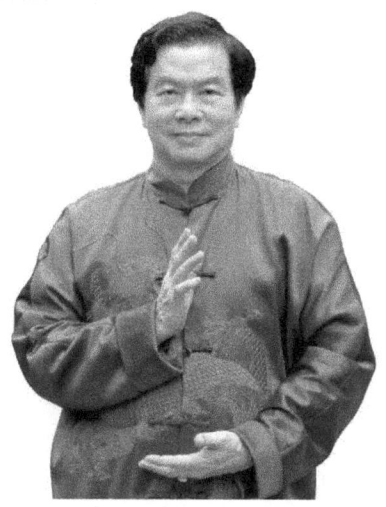

by Master Mantak Chia, the best-selling author of
Taoist Secrets of Love and *The Inner Smile*

'Emotional Detox through Bodywork, A Woman's Guide to Healing and Awakening'.

This is the book to heal and awaken the womanhood in you. I have had the experience of meeting Mal and have been very interested in his work ever since. And I'm grateful for his ability to help his clients surpass a state of survival into a state of celebrating life.

This book is full of information to rewrite your biochemistry for harmonious and joyful living. This book is the tool that you need to create the experiences you want in your life.

Mal Weeraratne

Women have been subjected to various misfortunes over the centuries and in the current times where they have become vehicles of agony. Mal has worked with over 3000 women from all over the world spanning across U.S, Europe, U.K and Asia. And having recognized the dire need of healing therapy required to reconstruct women, he took the initiative to start his brainchild, Tantric Journey School of Healing and Awakening.

Tantric Journey School of Healing and Awakening teaches the British pioneer therapy called 'Tantric Journey Bodywork'. Bodywork is an artisan-ship crafted with years of I research, teachings and validations by masters of the art in order to apply the healing massage techniques that bring about Emotional Detox.

This book encompasses the essence of Emotional Detox through a Tantric and Tao manner for women to awaken the goddesses that lie within them. Mal has mastered the art of Emotional Detox for a happier living by devising techniques to address the root of the problem in order to eliminate further proliferation.

If it's your desire to live a life free of your fears, past and pain, 'Emotional Detox through Bodywork, A Woman's Guide to Healing and Awakening' is the key to unlocking the great secret of a happier life. A few pages into this book and you will be welcomed to a world of loving healing and energy.

Acknowledgements

With a grateful heart, I must acknowledge my greatest teachers, the 3,000 plus female clients who came to me from all walks of life. I was a dedicated student to each and every one of them. I observed with curiosity and learned to fine-tune my skills with spirit and passion.

I am deeply indebted to the following teachers who showed me the path and enabled me to pioneer my deeply healing emotional release Bodywork:

- Charles and Caroline Muir – Tantra Yoga lineage
- Dr. Jack Painter – Dr. Wilhelm Reich lineage
- Grandmaster Mantak Chia - Tao Lineage
- Aunty Margret – Kahuna lineage
- Margot Anand – Osho lineage
- Brandon Bay – Self-healed cancer survivor

Special thanks to Shirley Turner, Hester Seddon, Roxy Grainge, Andrea Evans Charrington, Maya Fiennes, Humphrey Sherwood, Zeyana Haniffa, Hashini Nanayakara, Amer Amin, Kytka Hilmar and Dr. Tara Long, all who provided me with valuable support to make this journey a success.

Finally, my heartfelt thanks to my late father George Weeraratne, my wife, Sam Wimalaweera and twin boys, aged 14, and my two grown daughters Dr. Rebecca Wilson and Ramaine Wilson who support my often controversial work unconditionally and with complete understanding, acceptance and love.

Dedication

This book is dedicated to anyone who has suffered trauma either as a child or adult and is now seeking healing and awakening for greater freedom, connection, empowerment, love, peace and happiness. This book is also dedicated to all men who want to help their loved one to depart from her state of suffering and support her in her journey to attain healing.

Keep up to Date with New Releases

Thank you for getting a copy of Emotional Detox -A woman's Guide to Healing and Awakening through Bodywork- New Transformative Trauma Release Technique.

I'd like to offer you the chance to stay up-to-date on new book releases and courses with free access to my newsletter and a chance to download a free chakra chart.

By joining my newsletter you will be taking a big step towards improving your physical and emotional wellbeing. My newsletters are packed with self-help tips, news articles and updates plus exclusive offers and invitations.

Just visit http://www.tantricjourney.com/newsletter-sign-up and get instant access to the free chakra chart and start receiving the Tantric Journey newsletter today!

Preface

I was born with an innate ability to massage. Even at five years of age I enjoyed giving hand and foot massages and gained immense pleasure from the feel good factor that I could bestow on others. I was not trained at first, but I enjoyed the art of massage and it was as natural to me as breathing. It is impossible to describe how good it feels to give a really good massage to someone and feel them relax and respond.

There are so many different types of massage and I fully embrace this amazingly broad world. I believe that you evolve as a therapist and that deep in-depth knowledge is gained through experience. You never stop learning in this field as you continually adapt and adjust your technique. Massage is so much more than just a collection of techniques; if administered by an experienced therapist it is an empowering, practical and beneficial treatment.

Whilst I never stopped massaging, it wasn't until my wife took over a beauty salon that I decided to pursue a career as a therapist. In the beginning I gained such satisfaction when a client enjoyed their treatment, but then a few clients experienced an adverse reaction to my Bodywork. This was a frightening experience for both me as a therapist and for the client as she underwent what is commonly called, 'healing crisis'. I couldn't understand what I was doing wrong, so I embarked on a quest to discover why my female clients were experiencing trauma after deep tissue massage and followed my impulse to understand women and their emotional blockages.

It was my hunger for knowledge that led me to travel around the world and learn under the tuition of various pioneers and experts and eventually after years of training I became the first Certified Tantra Educator in the UK, from Source School of Tantra (USA).

My work is all about helping people to gain release from negative trauma and transform their life, allowing them to cast off negativity and emerge like a butterfly from a chrysalis. I believe that women hold great capability for overwhelming joy and, put simply, my work removes emotional blockages that stop the embodiment of this joy.

Yoni massage (pronounced, YO-NEE - the Sanskrit word for the vagina), is a therapy which can sometimes push your boundaries because it is capable of releasing oceans of tears, anger, mistrust and other emotions connected with our pain – both physical and mental – but it can also release great laughter, joy and deep pleasure which can in turn produce a heightened state of awareness. A Tantric Yoni massage can enable you to become aware of your creative feminine energy. This energy is very powerful and sometimes you are not ready for it, so you can feel confronted by all sorts of obstacles. But with a certain determination and willingness to be healed, you can push those boundaries and have a beautiful break-through. These experiences are not just ecstasy-like states, they are highly spiritual.

Because my treatment methods challenge many of the fixed ideas society holds about how female sexual dysfunction should be treated, it is only natural that I met much opposition over the course of my learning, treating and teaching career in the Tantra sector. Opposition will always be there as my work is ground-breaking and hard for even medical professionals to comprehend. I am never upset by opposition and resistance to my work as I am aware that it is nothing personal, it is simply that many people have never experienced my work or heard about it before and they even do not have the capacity to understand it, due to the culture and religious belief systems we are living in.

It is not unusual for pioneers in their field to encounter opposition, ridicule and even persecution for their views. Creating a new paradigm for helping women was always going to be difficult in this arena. However, I strongly believe that we no longer need to be restrained by the limitations of treatment imposed by the cultural traditions of the "traditional woman" which was the expected model or standard for females prior to the late 20th century (and a standard that continues to exert influence for many men and women today). Nor do we need to react with guilt, shame, or hostility when the nature of a new treatment makes you feel uncomfortable, after all, new philosophies and treatment are nearly always viewed with suspicion. Take for example Galileo; his work on astronomy made him famous and he was eventually appointed court mathematician in Florence. His work was ahead of his time and in 1614, Galileo was accused of heresy for his support of the Copernican theory that the sun was at the centre of the solar system. This was revolutionary at a time when most people believed the Earth was in this central position. In 1616, he was forbidden by the church from teaching or advocating these theories. We now of course recognise the merit of his work, but he was branded a deviant. In 1632, he was again condemned for heresy after his book 'Dialogue Concerning the Two Chief World Systems' was published. This set out the arguments for and against the Copernican theory in the form of a discussion between two men. Galileo was summoned to appear before the Inquisition in Rome. He was convicted and sentenced to life imprisonment, later reduced to permanent house arrest at his villa in Arcetri, south of Florence. He was also forced to publicly withdraw his support for Copernican theory. Being unorthodox does not always lead to popularity and recognition, but without those willing to work outside of accepted theories and practices then we would never see any progress and advancements made in history.

Undoubtedly the biggest challenge I face in my work is that the majority of women have been abused by men and often this abuse has taken place in the yoni. As a male healer, women initially feel resistance in allowing me to treat them. Many of my clients have been victims of sexual assault by men and as a result they experience feelings of hostility towards men as well as a deep rooted fear of men. Working with women who have trust issues, many of whom tell me that "they cannot bear to be touched", is a huge undertaking, but what is remarkable is the transformative healing that all of my clients go through.

The one constancy in my life has been that my commitment to my work has remained unshaken, for I have seen the deeply healing and life- changing effects my work has on my clients. The belief I have in my work has encouraged me to keep going in the face of adversity, but moreover, it has been the faith and gratitude of over three thousand female clients from around the globe that has given me the strength to continue my work.

I hold gratitude to all my clients for their loyalty and support for my work; I have learned so much from each of them. Each time I treat a new client I learn something new. My knowledge is continually expanding and, having treated over three thousand women from around the globe, I have been offered a unique insight into human sexuality since 1994. This level of practical experience combined with training and a lot of research has resulted in me holding a wealth of knowledge that I now wish to share with men and women. In this desire lies the manifestation of this book and the creation of my training school, called Tantric Journey School of Healing and Awakening.

Introduction to my Work

Everyone experiences some form of trauma at some stage in their life. For many people the impact of trauma has long lasting effects and leads to post traumatic coping strategies which include:

1) struggles with fragmented memory;
2) dismissal or minimisation of the trauma;
3) self-blame for violence and abuse:
4) a deep felt sense of uncertainty etc.

These negative themes resonate strongly into our expressions, feelings, thoughts, actions, responses and the decisions we make and often we remain unaware of the root cause of our anguish, pain and bad decision making.

The reason for my work, as I see it, is to help individuals get past a state of survival and to live a life of celebration. Many of my clients initially talk about simply "getting through the day". They describe how they encounter a reoccurring sense of being emotionally and physically drained and that each day sees them "running on empty" and that after performing basic functions they feel spent and so depleted that they have nothing left to give to tasks outside of the daily rituals of essential being. They are not living, but only surviving.

My belief is that surviving in life is not enough. Life is supposed to represent more than just an existence. Our lives are meant to be joyous and rich, and each day should end with a feeling of gratitude for more moments to celebrate and remember. We should close our day feeling accomplished and refreshed, happy and relaxed. Emotional blockages form from emotional traumas throughout life. In my work, I help individuals clear these blockages and subsequently improve the quality of their lives.

In order to treat those affected by emotional blockages, trauma and those who feel ill at ease, I have developed a unique treatment plan called Tantric Journey. This treatment will be explained fully within the chapters of this book, but it is sufficient to say, that over twenty years of study and practical application of ancient, and modern practices have resulted in pioneering work and astounding results.

After being treated with Tantric Journey my clients find themselves free of symptoms and discomfort. They find their direction by attuning themselves to their inner needs. They find freedom from negative patterns through deep clearance and balance. Modern research reports back up these results. When we are first born, we are free and pure, filled with positivity and love, which is the true essence of our being. Throughout our lives we add layer upon layer of negative beliefs, conditioning, and emotions as a result of physical and psychological abuse. The body harbours these negative emotions and traumas as a result of dismissing and bottling up and releasing them as and when they occur to only cause distress. This leads to blockages in our body's energy system which results in "body armouring," which I will explain fully within this book.

How trauma registers and accumulates within the body is best described by Dr. Peter Levine in his ground-breaking book 'Waking the Tiger': Healing Trauma. In it, he discusses his observations of animals in the wild, and how they deal with and recover from life-threatening situations. He concludes that their behaviour gives us "an insight into the biological healing process," and that "the key to healing traumatic symptoms in humans lies in our being able to mirror the fluid adaption of wild animals" as they avoid traumatisation in reacting to life-threatening situations.

It is true that in the jungle, animals experience many more traumas in each and every moment; however animals are not subject to blockages. They remain healthy and we see no signs of depression, obesity, cancer, and other such illnesses.

My personal work has been a journey of discovery and a study of this process where I act as a guide to help my clients find equilibrium. Through this journey, I unearth what individuals are truly needing out of their lives and relationships. Based on client feedback from the three thousand plus women I have worked with over the years, I have been told that my approach is practical, compassionate, and honest.

Perhaps this is due to the fact that I view the client as the expert in their experiences, and myself as the expert in interventions to be used to gain optimal functioning and performance in life.

Over the years, I have synthesized my work, my experiences, and my training to develop my speciality, which I refer to as the Tantric Journey. I am pleased to offer my clients a path to empower themselves. I value my work and see it as an honour to perform the work I do with others.

Throughout the years, my clients have enjoyed the many benefits of the Tantric Journey, which often incorporates the following goals:

- To help with sexual dysfunctions and to enhance Sexuality: to be an Orgasmic being;
- To get rid of body armouring and tension in order to soften the hardened body tissues and to promote relaxation; to learn to completely let go;

- To remove negative imprints, memories, emotions, blocks, conditioning and beliefs that have been held for many years around sexuality, and to make you feel more open and positive;
- To help remove aches, pain and numbness and to improve sensitivity, pleasures and sexuality;
- To help with many stress-related conditions such as depression, frustrations, insomnia;
- To help deal with issues around sexuality and sexual identity;
- To improve relationships and help finding a soul mate;
- To be able to stretch your boundaries at your own pace;
- To be awakened and be connected with your own divine self in a safe, caring, loving environment, within your own sacred space;
- To ease or remedy low self-esteem and timidity;
- To help with drugs, alcohol and other dependency issues.

Through the advanced Tantric Journey practices, I've been able to help my clients experience all seven levels of Altered States of Consciousness to help them heal their body, mind and spirit from past traumas.

I've found that before meeting with me, clients are hesitant about using these practices to heal the mind, body, and spirit. In general, Tantra is completely misunderstood in the west. Tantra is a very ancient science and a philosophy; however, many modern concepts of what Tantra is have taken away its real meaning. I use the name Tantric Journey for my treatment because it stops people making judgements about the treatment before exploring its true nature, also Tantric Journey incorporates other holistic practices such as yoga therapies and talking therapies. Tantra means expansion, and the journey is the journey into an expansion. It is not my journey to take; it is the client's individual journey that I am willing to take with them.

My female clients come from all different walks of life and from all over the world as the list below demonstrates:

1. Royalty and Titled Aristocrats
2. Celebrities and actresses from Hollywood
3. Models and beauty queens from all over the world
4. Singers, musicians and dancers
5. All scales of educational achievement from those with PhDs and degrees to those with no formal education
6. Wealthy and successful
7. Poor or in financial difficulty
8. Professionals and Business women
9. Leading all types of careers from Lawyers, Gynaecologists, medical doctors to massage therapists
10. Prostitutes, Lap dancers and Escort girls
11. Nuns
12. Tantric Dakinis and other spiritual women
13. My clients range from married, to separated, single parents and singles
14. The age range of my clients is from 18 to 80 years
15. Able and disabled (where I visit)
16. Heterosexuals, bisexual and lesbians
17. All nationalities, races, religions, cultures from USA, UK, Europe, Australia, Asia and the Middle East

Each with her own personal traumas, emotional blockages, and experiences. Usually, my clients come to see me for one or more of the following reasons:

1. They don't want anyone to know that they have a problem with their love, intimacy or sexuality.
2. All famous and well known clients fear tabloid newspapers getting their story and the journey to see me is a secret and only through word of mouth.

3. They don't want to evoke their partner's insecurities, a position that makes the process twice as difficult unless the partner is willing to collaborate and participate on the healing journey.
4. They find it impossible to share their past with their partner, close relatives or closest friend.
5. There are also some instances when women don't know why they are blocked, as the past events and memory is in the subconscious mind. So women find it difficult to explain why they want to come and see me.

My aim is to illustrate in this book, how Tantric Journey is a transformational treatment for awakening, sexual healing and relationship therapy. It doesn't matter what your beliefs are, where you're from, or what traumas you've experienced; Tantric Journey is a healing voyage, where you can open up your mind, body, and heart to all the healing power of love.

Throughout this book you will be learning the principles that have guided me and made my life a success by overcoming all obstacles in life. Each chapter has a lesson, followed by my story and finally a request to join the discussion to share your story and join the conversation. I want to open the door to you, the reader. I want to offer you an invitation to join ......

"Trauma is hell on earth. Trauma resolved is a gift from the gods."
- Dr Peter A. Levine

Tantric Journey Bodywork for emotional release is my passion. Freeing women from the blocks which keep them from fully experiencing their own life force is a big claim, but I have repeatedly found that it is actually possible. It is not easy, it is not always quick, but it is in essence a simple process and the results for thousands of clients show that the transformation and opening to life that they experience is a precious gift. I'm excited to share my knowledge and Tantric Journey with you.

Defining A New Transformative Healing Technique

Tantric Journey is a revolutionary healing technique that has been developed over a number of years to combine Eastern and Western knowledge, blended with ancient and modern wisdom creating a transformative healing technique that facilitates emotional, physical and spiritual restoration. Tantric Journey is a catalyst for:

1. The release of both emotional and physical toxins from the body
2. Enhancing love, intimacy and sexuality
3. Improving relationships
4. Healing the body, mind and spirit

The Four keys of Tantric Journey are:

1. Deep Bodywork to evoke emotions and to relax the body
2. Deep breathing to release evoked negative emotions
3. Sounds to disperse emotions through expression
4. Body movements to disperse stagnant negative emotions and to make way for the positive emotions to flow freely

Tantric Journey is an awakening and healing process based on the principles of Tantra and Tao amongst other wisdoms.

Questions about this Book

Isn't Tantra about Sex?

This is a very common misconception. Tantra explores all of the energy centres or Chakras in the body, including the Second Chakra that is associated with sexual energy. Tantra treats all the Chakras with an equal amount of time and consideration. We will explore the meaning of Tantra in more detail in the course of this book but, in short, Tantra is about nothing and everything, not just sex. Tantra explores sexual energy as an aspect of life and as a result it is more strongly linked with sexual energy than other traditions.

In summary Tantra is about: Trust, Sexuality, Intimacy, Love, Communication, Vision and Spirituality.

What about all those Tantric Massages I see offered on the internet?

Websites that offer 'Tantric Massages' that are filled with erotic suggestive pictures of the masseurs are generally not practising Tantric healing. Often sensual massage will be couched in "Tantric" language which, much to the dismay of true Tantra teachers, has become a bi word for erotic massage.

These erotic massage parlours are simply borrowing the name of Tantra to give their services a touch of Eastern flavour and this is not a true reflection of Tantric practices.

What about all those courses that explore sexual energy I see advertised?

There is a demand for courses that explore sexual energy and these courses often concentrate on the Second Chakra and on sexual pleasure. There is a ready market for these types of courses and they are often misleadingly branded as "sexual healing". Sadly this reduces Tantra to just a set of sexual techniques that does not explore all the energy centres or teach how to integrate them.

What is Tao?

I had the honour to study with one of the world's foremost contemporary Taoist masters, Mantak Chia and incorporate Tao practices into my unique therapy blend known as Tantric Journey.

Both Tantric and Taoist principles consider sexual energy as the same as life force, and both practices use the energy centres of the body to increase life force as a means to increased spirituality and improved health and longevity.

I will explain more about these modalities further on in this book.

Is this book suitable for women who have been sexually abused?

Yes, many women have experienced sexual abuse at some stage in their life and many of my clients come to me to resolve issues that are linked to their experience of sexual abuse.

Crime statistics do not accurately reflect the level of sexual abuse or invasion that exists as often these events go unreported. These experiences often occur during childhood and may even have been at the hands of a family member or family friend. It is often not just the trauma of the abuse that is damaging to the child but the sequence of events that ensue, including: not being believed, fear, shame, betrayal, medical examinations, official interviews or being trapped in a pact of secrecy with the abuser.

In addition to sexual abuse there are many other experiences that can cause sexual trauma in a woman and examples of these are being judged by family, friends or peers for early sexual explorations or being branded as promiscuous and feeling 'dirty' or 'used' as a result that in turn leads to a sexual shutting down.

When a woman encounters a sexual experience that she finds traumatic her energy system freezes and in many cases this freeze is so effective that the woman supresses all memories of the traumatic event. The trauma is locked with her and trapped in her cellular memory. A woman who is supressing sexual trauma in her body is unlikely to enjoy sex or experience full orgasms, though she may have no idea why this is. However, other women who retain trauma around their sexuality engage in unconscious sexual acts, veiling the feelings of guilt, shame and inadequacy.

Many of the thousands of clients I have treated in my practice have experienced sexual abuse and this sort of trauma cannot be dealt with by talking therapies alone because the trauma is trapped in the body and not the mind. (I will address the mind/body connection later on in this book). Countless female clients have described feelings of sexual numbness or have described how penetration is painful and distressing. Through their treatment sessions with me these women have felt the return of feelings -- although I always warn that the Tantric Journey healing path can be painful for everything that was not felt when the trauma occurred will be felt physically and emotionally as part of the healing process.

The Silent Epidemic

Our bodies are made like an onion, with layers of emotions stored from the time we are conceived, with all our life's experiences being collated and stored in our cellular memory. It is as though our body is like a gel and within it; every part is electrically and energetically connected.

Physical - Emotional Body

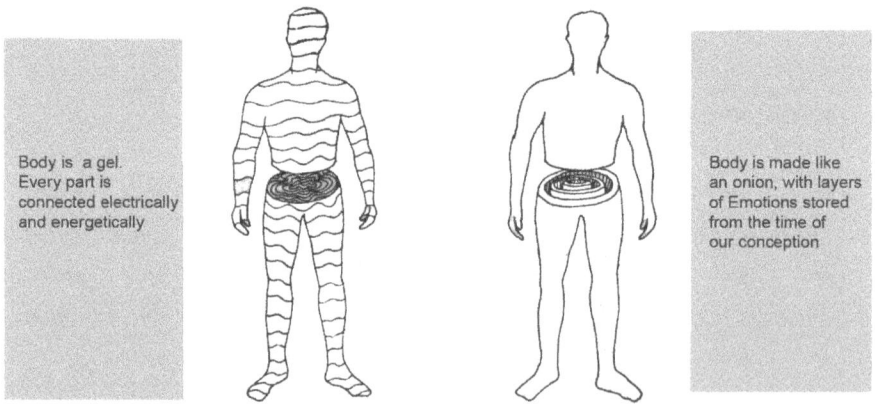

Body is a gel.
Every part is
connected electrically
and energetically

Body is made like
an onion, with layers
of Emotions stored
from the time of
our conception

Emotions are stored in our myofacia tissues in three levels
Skin, extrinsic muscles and intrinsic muscles

As we progress through life, we are continually subjected to a learning process to survive. Information we process gets stored in our cellular memory which is a great resource to us because it means that we can call upon experience as in the phrase, 'you never forget how to ride a bike'.

Whilst positive memories are catalogued in the cellular memory, trauma and abuse are also stored in the cells. However, when we have traumatic or abusive experiences, if we do not have the necessary consciousness, resources, or support available to process them, these experiences are stored in a raw or unprocessed form and can become emotionally and physically toxic.

We may not remember a source of trauma in the conscious mind, but the cellular memory will react to the trauma as if the trauma is raw. An example of this is if you have ever had someone touch part of your body and experienced an uncomfortable emotional response that was not consistent with the present or the situation. Cellular memories or unprocessed events can arise for you to make sense of and resolve or heal at any time; the problem is that often you won't know how to process these stored emotions. Tantric Journey excels at helping an individual in all aspects of the release process: allowing the negative stagnant emotions, as a result of the cellular memory to surface, supporting conscious exploration, releasing and letting go whilst holding the space and providing the safety to let go.

What I mean by releasing cellular memories is not forgetting about or erasing bad memories, but about transforming the raw cellular imprints into something that is processed and ultimately released. Tantric Journey supports the client accessing and releasing the memories and the consequences to your inner state of being. This is often a traumatic and dynamic process, which requires the guidance of a qualified and experienced healer to enable quick and effective release. There are other options, for example a life-long pursuit of a spiritual path, yoga or meditation, but these will take longer to achieve results.

One of the quick options relied on in the West is the prescription of drugs to suppress the emotions or to numb the pain. This option will not get rid of the emotion that is causing the symptoms, but will instead provide temporary comfort.

Another option is to remove the symptom by surgery. Surgery does not remove the core emotions causing the symptom, but does buy the patient some time to do something about the root of the problem; however, if nothing is done, research has shown that the symptoms will return often from a different site in the body.

The most popular form of treatment in Western culture is to receive Talking Therapies such as counseling and psychotherapy, which may help to a certain degree as the mind communicates to fix the body. However, I find when a client is subjected to trauma, she normally disassociates herself from the body by disconnection between the mind and body. In this situation communications to the mind cannot reach the body due to body and mind disassociation.

Talking therapy will serve best with a person whose body and mind is well connected. On the other hand a person who is so well connected can heal themselves with no external help by using their own self-healing mechanism.

In contrast, Tantric Journey directly contacts the deeply-rooted emotion in the body's cellular memory and helps remove it.

Tantric Journey is helpful in all the stages of recovery and will bring you back in touch with your purity and sexual aliveness. It is a worthwhile process that enriches and rewards the life of those that decide to embark on the process.

Either from physical or emotional sources things which we store within our bodies can become toxic. Within the physical realm, we store toxins from what we eat, drink, breathe and consume in terms of stress levels, lifestyle and our physical surroundings. Within the emotional realm, we store toxins from our belief systems, physical abuse, psychological abuse, sexual abuse, illness, trauma, shock and so forth. Some examples of childhood traumas can include:

- Parents separation or divorce
- Change from breastfeeding to bottle feeding
- Accidents and injury
- Sexual, physical and psychological abuse (66% of females and 33% of males in the UK)
- Religious and cultural beliefs to act against nature
- Medical examinations, operations, circumcision
- Exposure to natural and manmade disasters
- Death of a loved one
- Exposure or seeing violence and trauma happening to others in real life or in a film, video game, newspapers on television or in another media form.

This forms any combination of the following and stores them in our cells: sadness, insecurity, fear, rejection, shame, rage, guilt, greed, ego, mistrust, abandonment, anger, frustration, jealousy, disgust, contempt and spite.

As we grow, these stored emotions of childhood trauma cannot remain buried. Eventually we see signs manifesting; for women, this commonly includes:

- Loss of libido
- Self-harming
- Submissive behaviours
- Self-blaming
- Sexually shutting down

In men, these are typically manifested as follows;

- Aggression
- Violence

- Destructive behaviours
- Blaming others
- Controlling behaviours

The law of Physics states that energy cannot be destroyed, it can only be transformed.

Tantric Journey Philosophy states that all goals in life can be achieved with pure energy: being able to transform negative emotions, feelings, thoughts and actions into positive.

The Journey

In my broadest definition, I view symptoms of depression, anxiety, panic, addictions, sexual dysfunction and perversion as indicators of unresolved experiences that cause us to develop erroneous beliefs about ourselves, and store negative emotions in our cells. People logically know that the disturbing event is long gone, but cannot seem to reconcile it or aren't even aware that the adverse event has caused the memory to be harboured in their cellular memory.

I only work on female clients because I believe working on the opposite polarity gives the best healing results. When men and women are perfectly aligned they are the opposite energies of each other. The feminine is the force of life and source of inspiration. The feminine moves in all directions while the masculine moves in one direction. The feminine needs the masculine to give it direction, focus and resolution, whilst the masculine needs the energy of the feminine to give it motivation and passion. The masculine and the feminine need each other to be balanced and the cohesion created is like the Yin and Yang that represent duality forming a whole. In Tantra masculine is defined as Shiva or pure consciousness while the feminine is defined as Shakti or pure energy.

Whilst it is ideal for a man to heal a woman and a woman to heal a man because of the opposite polarities, is it possible for a therapist to be the same gender? Yes, but the therapist would need to activate their opposite energy. For example, a woman can heal a woman by using her masculine energy and a man can heal another man by using his feminine energy.

Most women have been hurt and damaged by men, starting with their closest family members, and then by boyfriends, and husbands. It's not only sexual abuse but physical, psychological and verbal abuse that will create trauma within the body. I must also add this trauma is not just in this life time, it could be ancestor's trauma that are stored in your cellular memory through the gene, which can go back to 1000s of years. Nevertheless ancestor's trauma plays only a very small % of our symptoms, while our childhood trauma from year 0 – 7 years plays the highest % of our symptoms.

Grief can also cause this trauma. The loss of a father in childhood can be a huge trauma for a young girl, who will then face a deficit of masculine love and affection. She will then experience feelings of abandonment and rejection which will then make it difficult for her to find the right partner or to stay in a long term relationship. She will continually be searching for 'Mr. Right', hankering after a lost love, or hanging on waiting to find 'The One' that will make her life complete or perfect. This quest to find the perfect partner is really a search to find the lost masculine love they have been deprived of, this deprivation is within them.

A trained Tantric Journey healer will be able to earn her lost trust in the masculine and hold the space for her to release negative emotions. This can help her repair old wounds and cultivate positive emotions which help her in many different ways in her life. These yin – yang polarities have been mentioned in the ancient Chinese texts as the best form of healing. This works the same way for men as they will benefit from a female healer rather than a male healer. It is usual behaviour to forget about childhood abuse as it is the mind's way of protecting itself. Some psychologists believe that forgetting childhood sexual abuse is a deep-seated unconscious blocking out of the event, an involuntary mechanism that automatically keeps painful memories out of consciousness.

In their recent study, Clancy and McNally detail how child sexual abuse victims can forget without trying, showing how this is a normal protective reaction. However, they go on to detail how victims feel that, despite not knowing of their abuse, once memory recovery had taken place, they "related their abuse to a history of later drug and alcohol problems, food abuse and gambling; others felt that the experience cut them off from other people. Most feel that the assaults affected all aspects of their lives. "It created a whole bunch of issues for me surrounding trust, intimacy, control and food, and other people. It's affected all my life. There's nothing untouched.". (The Trauma Myth: The Truth about the Sexual Abuse of Children - and Its Aftermath by Susan A. Clancy).

Clancy points out that "many researchers believe the trauma of the abuse is what causes the negative impact later in life. Research suggests that, in many cases, it may be the recall of the event and the retrospective interpretation of it, rather than the event itself, which causes the problems." It is true that the recall of these memories needs to be treated in a safe and trusting environment. Talking therapies alone will not resolve the emotional and physical scarring that the abuse has caused in the body.

One reason people don't talk about abuse is that they're not actually clear what it is, or that it's even happened to them. People don't talk about abuse whether it be physical, emotional or sexual because of fear, shame and the social taboos that surround the topic, whereas to others the details of the abuse are a blur, some are not clear what abuse is and others do not want to be labelled as a victim. The abuse is so painful that they disassociate themselves at the point of trauma.

At the centre of abuse is betrayal of trust and inability to give consent. Consent is a very important element and this is one of the healing aspects of Tantric Journey. Through this work sacred choice and consent are introduced.

I often treat clients who have been sexually abused at some stage in their lives and find it difficult to have regular orgasms with a partner or find it difficult to find a partner or to stay in a long-term relationship. Some have no recollection of any abuse, but still can't have regular orgasms. Most of my clients are referred to me by word of mouth and they understand the nature of my work to be emotional release through Deep Bodywork, yoni massage and female ejaculation, which I will talk about later on. They are of the understanding that my treatment programme will enable them to have regular, full body orgasms and to maintain a healthy and happy quality of life.

Expectations vary between clients. Some expect to have a full body massage with a yoni massage (Yoni (pronounced, YO-NEE) is the Sanskrit word for the vagina), during their first treatment; whilst others are not ready for a yoni massage, but enjoy a deep body massage. The yoni massage is not performed as a sexual act. Instead it is an affective form of Bodywork and de-armouring that can build trust and confidence between the giver and receiver as well as connect the receiver to her inner sensuality resulting in a feeling of complete well-being, happiness, fulfilment and contentment.

The purpose of the yoni massage is to relax the receiver and to bring her inner emotions to the surface so that she is free to shed negative emotions and express her natural, powerful, orgasmic being. The experiences and feelings that a woman may have during the yoni massage can be profound and wide reaching; ranging from anger, sadness, loneliness, sensuality, betrayal or happiness. The idea of a yoni massage is not to work to any pre-defined expectation but is simply to witness the receiver; holding the space for her whilst she heals and to honour and respect her feminine nature as a divine Goddess.

Long held hang-ups about sexuality and the shame and guilt associated with the sexual zones of the body have created deep-seated barriers that prevent people from fully expressing themselves. By the yoni being labelled a 'private part' it has created barriers and moral judgement on the merit of this area of work. When a woman receives a yoni massage it allows her to overcome these barriers and reconnect with her innermost core and deepest femininity. Yoni massage is not simply a hands - on massage technique, but instead involves the conscious direction of energy throughout the entire body through deep breathing, sound therapy and body movement.

The performing of a yoni massage gives women the ability to emotionally cleanse and energetically stimulate the Chakras (and physically stimulate hormone producing glands) as well as achieve emotional healing by releasing the traumatic pain held in the yoni. The yoni is not simply an area of sexual anatomy, but an important spiritual and energetic centre that is to be celebrated and embraced. Once a woman becomes in touch with her yoni energy, her connection to the whole of life is restored to its natural equilibrium as she receives emotional healing through releasing traumatic memories held in the yoni.

My working practices are defined by each individual client. I will massage a client fully clothed or without clothes: it is their journey and they are in control and their decisions will be based on how emotionally shut down they are. I liken each layer of a client's clothes to represent a layer of emotions which they peel off during each session as and when they feel comfortable. I meet all my clients from where they are emotionally and work around them to meet with their expectations rather than my expectations. Ultimately, most of my clients expect me to help them learn to ejaculate and release long held stagnant emotions.

> *"Let yourself be open and life will be easier. A spoon of salt in a glass of water makes the water undrinkable. A spoon of salt in a lake is almost unnoticed."*
> *~ Buddha*

The reason they seek me out is because they exhibit some of the following common symptoms of sexual dysfunction: low self-esteem, drug abuse, depression, over-achievement, under-achievement, poor relationships with others, sexual shutting down, unable to find the ideal partner or sexual acting out. Over a number of sessions healing begins to peel away the layers of negativity which heightens the client's energy levels.

Most clients are very apprehensive when they first come to me for treatment, even when they come through word of mouth. Throughout their lives these women have learned that to survive life they need to shut down and close off their heart. They have thought that the best way to protect themselves and stand the best chance of survival in life is to become closed. Whilst they don't always make this decision consciously, when life teaches you that things are inconsistent, physically and emotionally, and that events are out of your control, shutting down seems like the best way to avoid pain, but it also shuts the person off from the pleasures in life and individuals often find themselves on the path to destruction.

The anxiety and uneasiness of a new client is to be expected, which is why I spend over three hours in the first session just talking and listening to the client. This gives an opportunity for me to explain the features and the benefits of the treatment and for her to ask me questions and to establish trust and connection.

My few hours of talking therapy help them to open up their mind and give me permission to open their body. I begin with teaching them some breathing techniques, body movement techniques, toning techniques (making sounds), pelvic exercises, guided meditations and so forth, to open them up prior to the massage. I also ask them if they have any areas they would like me to avoid. I always honour their request.

Even after their written consent, I ask for their verbal consent before I start on their first yoni massage. After I perform three hours of Deep Bodywork the client relaxes into a trance-like state, unwinding, letting-go and opening. They transform from being rigid as their stresses and trauma begin to melt away and as a result they will usually give me permission to do a yoni massage, knowing that they can change their mind at any point during treatment.

I also discuss diet, lifestyle, and thought-handling with my clients, and typically recommend a detox and an alkaline diet and exercise plan such as Jade egg exercises to strengthen the pelvic floor muscles, yoga and meditation to optimize results.

After the session, clients go into a deep process which is sometimes unbearable, which I call a healing crises, trauma release or Kundalini Awakening which I will talk about later on. I always text the clients (with their prior permission) after a session, to find out how she is getting on and she is welcome to contact me any time for help and support, as trauma release is not well understood by the mainstream.

The Root Cause Approach

Why is Tantric Journey such a ground breaking treatment?

One of the biggest social problems we are facing today is that we're distancing ourselves from our roots, including nature, extended family unit, marriage and children. As a result of trauma we are also distant from our own self due to disconnection and dissociation. We are a society that is often termed, 'cash rich, time poor', and in many respects this analogy is correct. In this modern environment we are forced to suppress our emotions in order to conform to political correctness, modern ideology as well as cultural, religious and legal protocols. This does not allow us to fully and freely process our emotions as and when they arise. Instead we suppress them and store them in every organ in our body to be dealt with at a later date.

Exactly when and where one becomes ill as a result of negative emotions cannot be accurately predicted and the extent of the damage of stagnant emotions may take years to develop into a condition like a cancer, dysfunction, or may erupt immediately in panic attacks, accidents or in response to certain stimuli, through one or more of our five senses of touch, vision, hearing, smell or taste. This is the reason for the way we feel from time to time.

Similarly, the modern culture of eating processed food and drink on the go makes us get used to unhealthy eating habits which stores physical toxins into every organ in our body. It is a combination of physical and emotional toxins stored in every cell that makes our body acidic, which is dangerous to our health. The human body thrives at a slightly alkaline pH of 7.35, but poor diet and stress can change the body's pH to an acidic one in which all sorts of parasites and disease can thrive. Most diseased states can't exist when the body's pH is alkaline; bacteria, viruses' cancer cells and fungi cannot take hold. A body full of fast foods, drugs, and empty calories will provide an acidic environment for parasites to block natural repairing mechanisms in our body by blocking our circulation, lymphatic system and our very own energy system.

Modern medicine, drugs, alcohol, smoking, gambling, unhealthy foods and drinks provide us with a way to comfort our pain by suppressing our toxins and numbing our body to sensor the pain and suffering. These choices also make our body develop a biochemical chain reaction, to depend on such external substances for our mere survival, thus creating a cycle of addiction and craving. Once a person can no longer find comfort from these substances alone; they go on to abuse themselves and / or others, to be violent and to be a silent virus in society by further damaging the innocent and vulnerable.

The main victims in this scenario are children who get abused and who grow up to be abusers themselves. They become available to be abused physically, emotionally and psychologically. The result of this vicious cycle is the inability to find a suitable partner, to maintain a lasting relationship, lasting career or even to stay in the same home and create a settled home life.

The way we feel, think, act and achieve as an adult is a by-product of our childhood trauma and daily dosage of our emotional and physical toxins. For our bodies to function healthily and our life to be successful in terms of good health, wealth and happiness, we need to store and circulate positivity energies such as happiness, pleasure, love, and kindness. Every positive success in our life is as a result of a positive wave of energy flowing from the base of our spine towards our head and out of our body, just like a full body orgasm. This enables us to reach our highest potential in a positive direction. What's blocking this positive energy flow and diminishing our success is the negative stagnant energies stored in our body such as fear, shame, anger, sadness, mistrust, greed, ego, rage, jealousy etc.

If we are able to surrender to all the negative emotions and detox our physical toxins from our body, there is nothing to block our positive energy flow. This is the key to enable us to achieve our highest potential.

Holistic Anatomy

The human body is a beautiful and complex creation, whereby trillions of cells all perform their different roles to formulate an integrated whole. It is easy to forget the connections between body, mind and spirit, yet everything in the body is intrinsically interconnected and integrated.

Cells are often referred to as 'the building blocks of life' and these tiny organisms are what give the body structure, performing physical tasks with groups of cells joining together to form tissues and different tissues collectively forming organs. With all of the organs and supporting structures forming systems in the bodies, the body could be likened to a large institution with various departments all carrying out functions: protection, communication, recycling, commands, control, energy input, waste disposal, transport and production. If you think of your system as a busy institution, a bit like a communications office, it will stand to sense that your internal body is not a static entity; it is constantly changing and adjusting.

Whilst the body exists in a state of continuous change there is an internal balance known as homeostasis, which constantly measures and adjusts to keep the body in a state of equilibrium. Homeostasis is the Western way of explaining the Yin and Yang concept used within Taoism. Explaining the nature of change and of complementary opposites, for example: night (Yin) and day (Yang), female (Yin) and male (Yang). These opposites, weave in and out together, dancing in and out of balance together creating a wholeness and complete balance together. One cannot exist without the other. It is worth noting that in Western physiology homeostasis only refers to physical functions.

Life itself is constantly moving and changing and the chemicals in our bodies adjust to keep us at optimum health. Everything in our system needs to work together to keep us fit and healthy in both physical and emotional terms. In the Western scientific tradition we love to classify and separate things into individual pigeon holes and so we divide the functioning of the body into systems and analyse each one as an isolated entity. The skin, the skeleton, joints and muscles, the heart and circulation, the lymphatic system, the lungs, the gut, the kidneys and bladder, the nervous system and the reproductive system are all dealt with individually, however, it is important to remember that in reality all of these systems are connected and that they do not function alone.

Bodywork for Trauma

Psychotherapy and other talking therapies have been and continue to be the first form of treatment for survivors of sexual abuse and for those with deep-seated emotional impairments. Whilst talking therapies are useful in the retrieval and integration of the disintegrated mind, there is another aspect to recovery: that of retrieving the body.

The body holds the scars of trauma and emotional release, therefore Bodywork is an effective method of treatment as it can access the trauma and releases it from the body – trauma is held in the body not the mind.

It is common for a traumatised person to resort to defensive coping mechanisms such as dissociation, with any future stresses resulting in tendency to escape through dissociation and a separation from awareness of the body's experience. While dissociation may temporarily serve an adaptive function, in the long term, lack of integration of traumatic memories seems to be the critical element that leads to the development of the complex behavioural change termed as Post Traumatic Stress Disorder.

The effects that trauma stored within the body has on regulation of bodily and emotional states is well documented. Chronic hyper arousal and attempts to adapt can lead to disturbances with sleep and digestion, eating disorders, and other forms of body distress. Survivors of abuse or childhood trauma are prone to experience depression and anxiety, and in some cases resort to self-harm to block out emotional pain.

Fragmentation of self, both in body and mind, increases vulnerability as the traumatised individual tries to navigate life with dissociated defences. This results in a gradual breakdown of defences, surfacing as problems in maintaining relationships, jobs, alcohol and substance abuse, or even suicidal thoughts.

As the body was integral to the trauma, it is also integral to the healing process. We now accept that the mind and body are interconnected. Interestingly, until the 1800s, most medical professionals believed that emotions were linked to disease and advised patients to visit spas or seaside resorts when they were ill. Gradually emotions lost favour as other causes of illness, such as bacteria or toxins, emerged, and new treatments such as antibiotics acted as 'cure-alls.

The connection between how emotional, mental, social, spiritual, and behavioural factors can directly affect our health is now once again a recognised modality and over the past twenty years, mind-body medicine has provided evidence that psychological factors can play a major role in such illnesses as heart disease, and that mind-body techniques can aid in their treatment. Clinical trials have indicated mind-body therapies to be helpful in treating chronic pain conditions. There is also evidence they can help to improve psychological functioning and quality of life; and with this growing understanding of body/mind connection, there has been increased interest and practice of providing Bodywork to facilitate wholeness. For some clients, after years of verbal therapy, there comes a time when they need and want to reclaim the body. This is where Tantric Journey Bodywork can help. Many women I see come to see me because they want to experience resolution at a deeper body level.

Emotional release through Bodywork provides touch and this is often something that my clients have been deprived of. Their trapped emotions from trauma have often left them with an aversion to touch and intimacy and the experience of touch is another important benefit of Bodywork. It involves learning that touch can be a pleasurable and positive experience and not just a source of pain and discomfort. Even for those clients I treat who are in a relationship, I find that many have difficulties with intimacy, receiving touch and feeling comfortable sexually.

When I treat a client I find a level of touch that is appropriate for each individual client. No two treatments are identical; everyone's treatment path is slightly unique. During a session I ask for their permission to perform Bodywork and clients can assume ownership of their bodies within this safe environment and determine their boundaries, having the ability to withdraw their consent at any stage. I have seen amazing transformations take place as a result of Bodywork as my work makes people empowered. People who cannot do or say anything to get out of a negative situation such as a physical or emotionally toxic relationship (because they are in a 'frozen' state), suddenly gain physical voice and empowered ability to take action and move away from negative people and situations.

Laura's Story – a real life account of a client's transformative experience

"When I was 18 I went off to university to study with high hopes of having a career in journalism. My family was so proud of me because I was the first person in the family to make it to higher education and I did feel a bit of pressure on me to succeed.

The first year away from home was fun and I certainly enjoyed the socialising part of student life, going out every weekend, drinking, socialising and yes partaking in casual sex. I never intended to have one night stands, they just sort of happened. I was struggling with the pressure of the course workload and was filled with a nagging feeling of insecurity about my abilities and also an overwhelming needy feeling. I turned to casual encounters as a way to express and satisfy my sexuality. I needed to take comfort in something and inspired by that old student adage, "drunk sex is better than no sex", I embraced one night stands whole heartedly.

I've always had a high sex drive and the thought of a cold empty apartment to go home to after a night out seemed to heighten my need for sexual partners. For brief moments my one night stand experiences were liberating and comforting, but afterwards I just felt numb and empty. I tried to bury my feelings of being a cheap hussy with delusions that I was just exploring my sexuality, but really I just wanted a partner and was secretly hoping that the sex would lead to something more serious. I was searching for security through human contact and was wanting all my other insecurities to wash away. To be fair the one-night-stands did temporarily wash away my feelings of despair and failure, but the next morning I always felt worse especially when the man left as whilst there was sexual fulfilment there was no emotional fulfilment.

Riddled with self-loathing, I labelled myself as a "slut", "slag" and "easy". Fearing that I would end up either pregnant or in an unsafe position from one to many casual affairs I decided to change my ways. I wasn't enjoying my course and I couldn't keep up with the work load. I decided to drop out of uni and go home. My one goal in life was now to find a partner and pop out a couple of babies. I wanted a simple life of home, children and benefits, after all this is what I had been raised to aspire to.

Within a week of returning home I had hooked up with a local lad and on the first date we went to bed and within a week we were living together. Life was temporarily bliss: I was pregnant, in the freshness of a new relationship and we had dreams for the future.

Things didn't stay blissful, now pregnant with my second child I felt trapped. My partner was controlling, selfish and aggressive. With outbursts of anger he would lash out at me, smash my belongings and use verbal abuse. I felt that I couldn't live with him but had no confidence to leave him.

Eventually with the support of my family I left my partner and started to live on my own with the two kids, but he still had control over me. Even after a year of living separately he still had emotional and physical control over me: calling me up when he wanted company, demanding my attention, emotionally blackmailing me into sex and even confiscating my car when I wouldn't do as he wanted. I didn't have the strength to escape his clutches and every time I saw him my words vanished, it was as if I had no power to fight back.

By chance I attended a talk with Mal about empowering your life and so much that he said made sense. I decided to go for three sessions with Mal and receive some deep healing therapy work and during these therapy sessions I went through some amazing transformations. During the session I felt an overwhelming sense of love and safety. There was physical and emotional pain during the initial session as I was releasing negative emotions held deep in my body including fear, shame and disgust. Following my treatment sessions I felt a sense of inner joy and happiness and for the first time in my life I knew who I was.

I stopped giving into the pressures of my ex-partner and had the strength to walk away from the negative and toxic situation completely. After my sessions I felt so alive and confident and I was finally able to find a loving supportive partner. I'm now looking forward to getting married and am running my own business, I will never forget the healing process I went through and am so glad I escaped the trap of the negative emotions I was holding within me."

Trauma and Natural Response

When a person experiences a traumatic event, such as, but not exclusively, sexual abuse, they often go into a "frozen state" whilst the abuse is going on as a way of 'surviving'. This is not a voluntary reaction; freezing is the best way the body knows to protect itself from the trauma of what was beyond its control. If fight and flight were not an option and the brain perceives death is imminent, it is the best way of protecting itself. In this state the victim of trauma enters an altered state of reality (a trance like state). Time slows down and there is no fear or pain. If harm or death does occur, the pain is not felt as intensely. This is a basic animal instinct and works on the premise that this response can increase chances of survival if the attacker (animal or human) thinks the person is dead.

The term 'fight or flight' has been recognised for a long time, whereas the state of 'freeze' has only recently been recognised as being applicable to humans. Fight or flight is all about hope and the chance of escape: it is focused upon survival through avoidance, and we activate it when we believe there's a chance we can outrun or fight off our attackers. The freeze response gets activated when we feel trapped and there's no hope: it is all about minimising pain.

So when escape is deemed impossible and fighting is not possible or the traumatic threat is prolonged, the limbic system can simultaneously activate the parasympathetic branch of the autonomic nervous system, causing a state of freezing called 'tonic immobility'. This is the same state that an animal caught as prey goes into; think of a rabbit freezing in the headlights. It is a natural survival instinct and the most basic of responses.

Arousal is controlled by the limbic system, which is located in the centre of the brain. This part of the brain regulates survival behaviour as well as emotion and memory. The limbic system has a close relationship with the autonomic nervous system (ANS). It weighs up a situation, signalling the ANS either to have the body rest or to prepare itself for strenuous effort. (The ANS has 2 branches: the sympathetic branch which is principally aroused in states of effort and stress, and the parasympathetic branch which is mostly aroused in states of rest and relaxation).

The freeze state prepares the body and mind for the worst; it allows them to endure the pain and still manage to lie perfectly still and stand the best chance of surviving the attack. When author Dr. Peter Levine, gives lectures on surviving trauma, he plays a video of a cheetah chasing a young impala. He is demonstrating to the audience exactly how the freeze response works. Predictably the cheetah catches the impala and it ruthlessly sinks its teeth into the young animal's neck and throws its lifeless body on the ground several times. It's an attack that is over in seconds. In this fearful moment the impala freezes and pretends to be dead, breathing stops for a moment, and sends out a smell of a dead animal. Then the cheetah sniffs the dead smelling impala and leaves it alone, stops the attack and walks away as predators like fresh meat and not dead animals. Then something miraculous happens, as the cheetah walks away, the impala comes back to life, as if wakening from a coma or hypnotic trance. You see the impala as it shivers all over and releases this 'survival' fear energy. The visible shaking and trembling is the completion of the survival process; it is letting go of the trauma before it stands up and runs away, making a clean escape. Animal biologists have concluded that if the animal did not complete the process and expel the trauma by shaking and trembling they would not survive the trauma.

For human beings, the freeze response is most likely to occur when we are severely scared and feel that there is little chance for escape and that we are unlikely to survive. It happens in instances of sexual abuse, rape, car accidents, torture and any situation that presents an imminent and horrific scale of trauma. Sometimes a person will black out, losing consciousness or freeze or mentally remove themselves from their bodies so that they don't feel the pain of the attack. This often leads to the victim having no explicit memories of the attack, but survivors of a freeze event will experience flashbacks and other (implicit) memory fragments from the storage of the negative emotions connected to the trauma that are stored in their cellular memory. These past emotional trauma shards will continue to impact and haunt the victim until the trauma is released from their system.

BURIED BUT NOT FORGOTTEN: HOLDING ON TO THE TRAUMA

This 'freeze state' also influences memory processing, which is why it may not be until well into adulthood that a victim remembers the incident, but just because they do not remember the incident does not mean that it is buried and forgotten, the trauma is held within the body where it is waiting for a trigger to come along and release the stored trauma. The negative emotions are like a volcano waiting to erupt and throughout the victim's life, the negative stored emotions bubble beneath the surface looking for a release. Often small spurts of negative emotion will be released without disruption or eruption, but instead culminating in negative, reactionary behaviour. Other times a trigger point will spur a major eruption and the trauma will be laid bare, leaving the survivor to interpret the feelings of abuse and process the effects of the past trauma that now encompass them.

It is important to understand that the trauma violated the victim's sense of safety and trust and reduced their sense of worth. In 2007 Van der Kolk studied the effects of experiencing trauma in childhood and he reported that it increased the survivor's levels of emotional distress, shame and grief, and increased their proportion of destructive behaviours. 'Destructive' behaviours included: 'aggression, adolescent suicide, alcoholism and other substance misuse, sexual promiscuity, physical inactivity, smoking, and obesity' (Trauma and Its Challenge to Society). Survivors of childhood trauma were also demonstrated to be more predisposed to have difficulty developing and maintaining long-term and meaningful relationships with caregivers, peers and marital partners. He also argued that adults with a childhood history of unresolved trauma were more likely to develop lifestyle diseases including heart disease, cancer, stroke, diabetes, skeletal fractures and liver disease whilst also being more likely to commit crimes and be involved with the penal system.

ADULT MANIFESTATIONS OF PAST ABUSE

Long-term effects of childhood sexual abuse are recognised as including depression, anxiety, and anger in adult survivors. But it is not just emotional responses to childhood sexual abuse that occur in women. Gynaecological problems, including chronic pelvic pain, dyspareunia (painful sex), vaginismus (tightening of vaginal muscles and closing the vagina), nonspecific vaginitis (infection such as candida or yeast infection or inflammation of the vagina), and gastrointestinal disorders have been diagnosed among survivors and linked by medical Doctors to incidences of past abuse.

This is because the past trauma is continuing to live inside the survivor's body. Emotion is energy in action that is designed to flow through our body. Strong emotions are important as they are the tools we use to create and shape our existence and how we interpret the world. These emotions are normal and healthy when they are flowing.

When our emotions are negative and stagnant as the result of trauma, this transfers to the body during the 'freeze' response; the body is like a storehouse of memory and every cell in our body responds to every thought, memory and experience we have. Continuous modes of negative thinking and the retention of negative emotions attached to past trauma memories will change and slow down the flow of emotion creating stagnant energy and producing body behaviours where disease will exist and advance. Holding on to negative emotions in the cellular memory will upset the chemical balance in the body causing physical and emotional distress to the sufferer.

TREATMENT AND RECOVERY

Because the 'freeze response' is controlled by the limbic system, brain stem, and spinal cord, talking therapies (such as counselling) tend to miss the areas where trauma and post-traumatic stress are to be found. Deep Bodywork and other somatic approaches are methods ideally suited to dealing with the core of trauma and releasing the pockets of negative emotion within the body, because they access our experience at a sensing and feeling level first, and verbally only as an important secondary process. It is important to understand that whilst the mainstream methods including counselling, marriage guidance or sex therapy have their merits, they are ineffective in these circumstances. Because emotions as a result of trauma are stored in the body and not in the head or in the mind they are unable to access and release the trauma in the way that Bodywork such as Tantric Journey can. Most traumatic experiences dissociate the person and disconnect the body and the mind. In this state, when you talk to the mind it cannot communicate to the body and it is for this reason that talking therapies alone may not fully resolve this type of trauma.

How does Deep Bodywork and Tantric Journey Access Trauma?

Tantric Journey is a combination of Deep Bodywork, Tantric practices and other holistic therapies that in combination have proven successful in the treatment of trauma. Treatment of trauma using Tantric Journey has reliably given results in the treatment of over three thousand women in the UK and Overseas.

To understand why Tantric Journey is so effective you have to firstly understand that trauma patients are trapped and frozen within space and time, encapsulated unconsciously by their past trauma. Because these survivors are in a deeply anxiety producing position, any use of touch is done extremely slowly and carefully. One of the characteristics of Deep Bodywork is its slow, sympathetic and sensitive application. This allows the trauma patient to engage his or her felt-sense and allows the trauma to be accessed.

Deep Bodywork in trauma related cases must be slow and sensitive in order to allow the client to process the trauma and for the stuck energy of trauma to be freed from the body. The process is to challenge the client from moment to moment during Bodywork, so she contracts and then to back off and give sacred space for her to expand. With each moment of contraction and expansion incorporating breath, you help her to release emotions and unwind.

It takes years of training and practice for a Tantra Practitioner to become skilled enough to safely access trauma quickly and efficiently. As this energy begins to free, typical manifestations in the clients' bodies can be trembling and shaking; followed by emotion, as the actual traumatic event gains access to the memory. During this process the practitioner needs to be experienced enough to 'hold the space' for their client and allow the healing process to take its course.

Through slow body work in a safe, sacred environment of trust and love, the client's capacity to remember, with the therapists support, increases. The client must trust the therapist before Bodywork can commence and eye gazing is an incredibly powerful technique that will help to connect the client to her true spiritual side and to trust the therapist and overcome initial feelings of vulnerability and overwhelming emotions. Eye gazing provides a direct soul connection removing barriers and creating connection and forging trust between client and therapist.

Tantric Journey Deep Bodywork evokes emotions embedded in body cellular memory. Deep breathing in through the nose and out through the mouth helps to disperse the evoked emotional and physical toxins from the body. While the inhalation is of one unit of air, exhalation should be seven units of air to facilitate the emotional release.

Life energy can also be increased through good sleep, exercise and eating patterns. A detox that involves avoiding alcohol and drugs is recommended. Whilst adopting a regular exercise routine boosts serotonin, endorphins, and other feel-good brain chemicals, it also boosts self-esteem and helps to improve sleep. Often changes in eating patterns are also recommended, eating small, well-balanced meals throughout the day will help you keep your energy up and minimize mood swings. Raw and fresh foods are recommended to help strengthen the immune system and flush the toxins from the body. Whilst you may be drawn to sugary foods for a quick boost or temporary feel good factor they provide, complex carbohydrates are a better choice with prolonged health benefits.

Relaxation techniques including meditation and yoga exercises are important elements of the re-building and healing process. These techniques provide rest and restoration for the mind and body and help to eradicate negative emotions stored in the body.

What Tantric Journey offers is not just a quick fix or wonder cure, but a highly effective combination of therapies resulting in one course of treatment that in skilled hands restores the equilibrium of the body and mind.

Body Armouring

Unfortunately, when sex has equalled pain (either physical or emotional), a vicious cycle often sets in and women avoid sex altogether or unintentionally put up barriers known as 'Body Armouring'. Dr. Wilhelm Reich, the pioneer psychotherapist and sexologist who postulated the orgasm theory, proclaimed that full orgasm is the very centre of human experience and ultimately determines the happiness of the human race. This means that traces of the emotional content of every sexual experience will be recorded in the muscular tissue of your genitals, including those from negative events or traumatic experiences.

Sexual abuse, rape, complicated childbirth; surgery or negative attitudes to sex may all contribute to the lack of ability to orgasm as every unsatisfied sexual experience is recorded in the cellular memory of your body.

Research has shown that only a quarter of women achieve orgasm through penile penetration, leaving three quarters in need of additional clitoral stimulation. It is estimated that twelve per cent of women are anorgasmic (never reach a climax). In fact because the sexual organs have been subjected to vigorous condemnation from childhood, onwards, the pelvic basin has become a major storehouse of negative imprints, restricting and inhibiting the woman's ability to enjoy full sexual capacity and preventing the full enjoyment of orgasmic release.

By creating an invisible body armour, your body is attempting to reduce its vulnerability to pain, discomfort and possible danger. In effect the armouring process not only protects from pain, but also from the woman's own desires and instincts.

Tantric Journey works to reverse the stored-up energy from traumatic events by using healing massages and breathing exercises. By working closely with my clients, I can ensure that they're able to effectively deal with the tragedies of the past in order to move onto the fulfilling relationships of the future.

Emotions Rooted
In the Body

Emotions may feel like they're governed by the heart or head, but there's a great deal of research that suggests emotions are rooted within our physical selves; that is, emotions are stored in every cell in our body's cellular memory. This means that traumatic experiences can be embedded deep within our bodies, which can only be released by undertaking deep, healing Bodywork such as Tantric Journey.

This is a fascinating field of study for many researchers, including Dr. Candace Pert, a pharmacologist and professor at Georgetown University. According to Pert, amino acid chains within the body help to connect emotions to the physical self; in other words, our amino acids, nerve endings, muscles, immune system and other body parts are all involved in a conversation that's dictated by our emotions.

Cell Receptors and Peptides

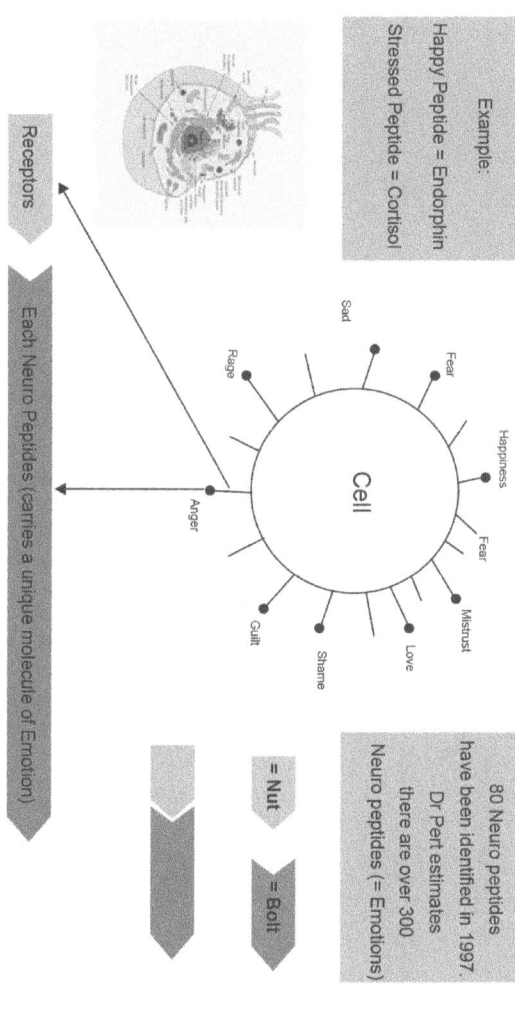

Example:

Happy Peptide = Endorphin

Stressed Peptide = Cortisol

Receptors

Each Neuro Peptides (carries a unique molecule of Emotion)

Sad
Fear
Rage
Happiness
Cell
Fear
Anger
Mistrust
Guilt
Love
Shame

80 Neuro peptides have been identified in 1997. Dr Pert estimates there are over 300 Neuro peptides (= Emotions)

= Nut

= Bolt

To realise just how critical emotions are to your physical being, try to remember your earliest memory. It's likely to be one in which you had a very strong emotional reaction to a stimulus. Perhaps you first remember your mother fearfully warning you to stay away from a hot stove, or the fascination you felt when you visited the zoo for the first time. Powerful emotions are so critical to our bodies that when we experience and recall them, they transform our physical selves. Good memories often produce happy and positive energy; memories from traumatic experiences can make the physical self feel ill or panicked.

Negative Emotions Feed Negative Thoughts and Actions
- Making us More Negative

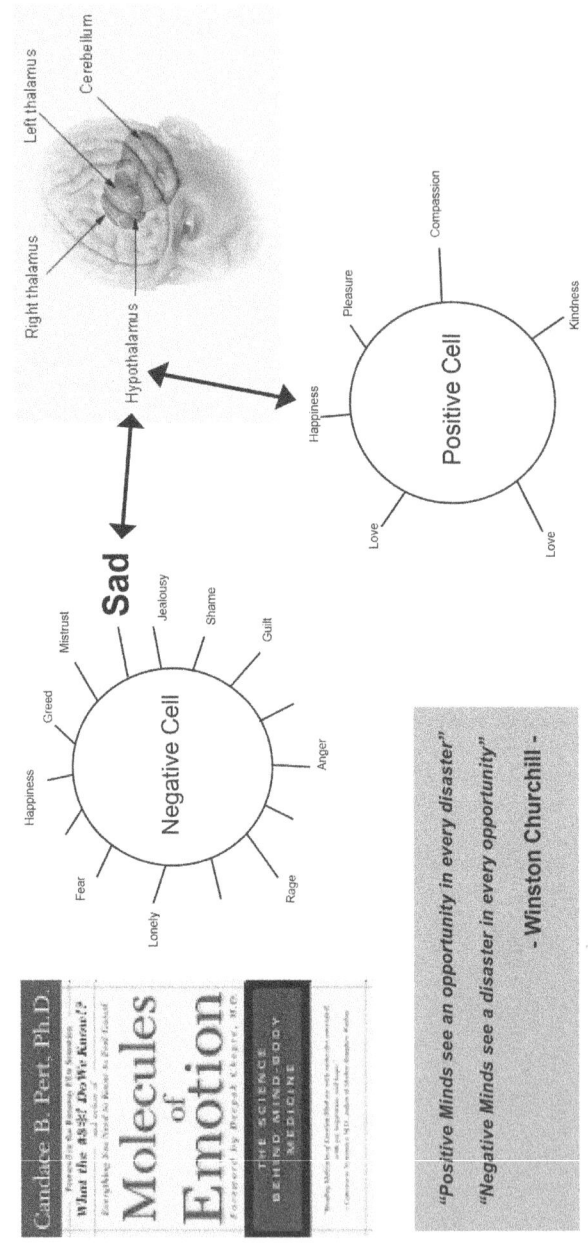

Dr Candace Pert, pioneering scientist and author of 'Molecules of Emotion – Why you feel the way you feel'.

Whether you're recalling good or bad memories, our bodies are programmed to be able to repeat the emotional experience, which can be accessed through the body in many ways. That means that emotions can't be fully expressed until they've reached your consciousness. This involves releasing the emotional energy at a cellular level before it can cause your body significant harm, as a great deal of research suggests that unexpressed emotions can be linked to physical illness.

In order to fully heal from a traumatic experience, it's important to release emotions stored within your body so that it can bubble all the way to the surface. When your emotions are integrated at higher and higher levels in the body, this allows your emotions to be brought into consciousness.

This is why one of the main healing techniques of Tantric Journey involves a deep tissue massage. The purpose of the massage is to relax, detox, tone, energize, and heal the body. It is important to treat the whole body holistically, as every body part is connected to one another.

To understand how deep tissue massage work, you should know that the body is made of the following four areas:

1. Pleasure areas
2. Emotional areas
3. Pain areas
4. Numb areas

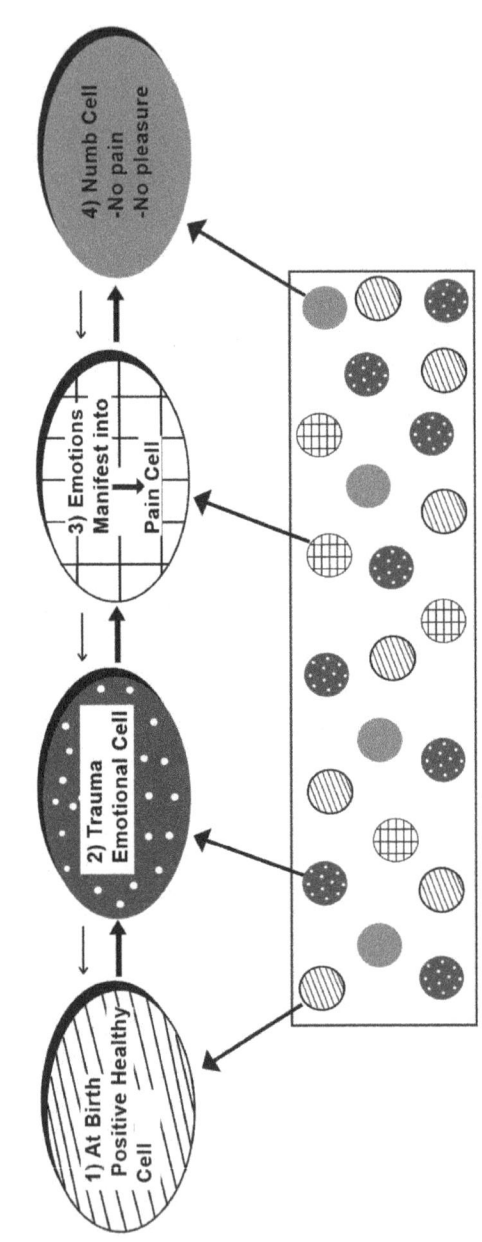

4 Points In The Body

1) At Birth Positive Healthy Cell

2) Trauma Emotional Cell

3) Emotions Manifest into Pain Cell

4) Numb Cell
-No pain
-No pleasure

When we're born, all of our bodies are made of pleasure areas; however, when traumatic events take place throughout our lives, these pleasure areas are turned into emotional areas. When these emotions are left repressed, these areas quickly become pain areas. This pain can be manifested as back and shoulder aches, headaches, and other manifestations. If you don't address body aches at this stage, body will then make such areas go numb.

This is the body's natural way of dealing with physical pain. The down fall of this is that you lose pleasure sensations from the body as well as pain, by shutting down. At this stage you may feel no physical pain, but due to shutting down your body, it may block your natural energy flow that promotes healing. This may lead to dis-ease, illness, dysfunctions, and so on.

A deep tissue massage works by transforming the numb area into pleasure areas again; but first, it's critical to go through the pain and emotions that might have been there for decades. During this massage, I remind my clients to breathe deeply to eliminate both the pain and emotional toxins from the body, thus promoting relaxation and healing. I also tell them to drink a glass of water before and after the massage to promote detox.

After a deep and emotional release massage, I always tell my clients that they need to find a peaceful, positive, and tranquil environment to be in, as this allows them to process the long-held emotions that have been trapped within their cellular memory.

Physical Detox: Replenishing your System through Alkalinity

For those of you familiar with basic anatomy and physiology, you may remember that our cells die and reproduce every couple years and you could be excused for thinking that when cells die so does the emotional memory that is stored within it; but sadly this is not the case. Negative emotions can transfer to new cells until the time that the emotional memories are released through emotional cleansing.

When undergoing healing through Deep Bodywork it is important to support your healing process by undertaking a physical detox. This is a good time to assess your eating habits and cravings. You probably know the term "gut feeling", well this derives from the fact that our guts are an emotional radar system: telling us when we're nervous, anxious, afraid, worried, happy, excited, in love and much more. When we don't feel confident with these emotions, many of us use food (or other things like alcohol, cigarettes, recreational drugs, etc) to crush our feelings.

Eventually it comes to a point where we've been crushing our feelings for so long we don't even know how we're feeling. We've become so numb we are disconnected from our pain and our digestive system is stifled. Hunger and cravings are two different things. Hunger is the body's way of making sure it is provided with energy, in the form of nutrients from food. When the stomach is empty, it releases the hormone ghrelin, which communicates with the brain's command centre, the hypothalamus. This creates the feeling of hunger and is how we know when to eat. Satiation of hunger is signalled by the release of the hormones leptin by fat cells, and insulin by the pancreas, in response to increased blood sugar. Cravings, however, are much more complex. Cravings are overwhelming sensation of desire for a certain food and are not connected to hunger. There are a number of chemicals in the brain that are associated with craving and to explore the science of cravings fully would require the space of a whole book, but one factor in craving for sugary or fatty foods is stress. When the body is stressed it produces a hormone called cortisol. The primary functions of cortisol are to increase sugar in the blood to be used up as energy by the body's cells, suppress the immune system and aid in fat, protein and carbohydrate metabolism. It also blocks the release of leptin and insulin which in turn increases hunger. This natural response is linked to a time in the history of man when stress was in response to danger and would necessitate energy being burned up during 'fight or flight'. Stress present in modern lifestyles causes the same bodily and emotional responses, though these days we are less likely to actually burn off the calories.

It is also worth noting that today's stresses and strains are often relentless and this means that the constant desire to reward ourselves for working long hours or perk ourselves up when we feel low has resulted in a sugar and fat rich diet in the West.

When dealing with emotional or physical pain we are also programmed to crave sugary foods as sweet food can actively alleviate pain by releasing opioids. Researchers at the University of Michigan found that chocolate causes the brain to release these euphoria-inducing chemicals. Whilst there is no harm in consuming high-fat and high-sugar foods from time to time, they should not form the basis of anyone's regular diet. The main issue is that fatty, processed and high sugar foods are acidic and an acid body is a magnet for sickness, disease, cancer and ageing. Eating more alkaline foods helps shift your body's pH and oxygenates your system. Alkaline foods keep your body healthy and functioning correctly, preventing and combating illnesses including cancer.

A surprising number and variety of physical problems and diseases can be caused by the problem of foods that are acid-producing after digestion. Both the modern lifestyle and diet promote acidification of the body's internal environment and in order to promote a healthy and functioning system it is important to address the acidity levels in your body.

A typical Western diet is currently composed mainly of acid-forming foods (proteins, cereals, sugars). Alkaline-producing foods such as vegetables are eaten in much smaller quantities, whilst acidifying stimulants including tobacco, coffee, tea, and alcohol are greatly consumed. Stress and physical activity (both insufficient and excessive amounts) also cause acidification.

Many foods are alkaline-producing or neutral by nature, but manufactured processed foods are mostly acid-producing and these are the ones that tend to be promoted in supermarkets and consumed for the benefit of convenience. It is essential to assess your eating patterns, for eating a diet that correctly balances acid and alkaline-producing foods is beneficial to health and vitality.

It is essential to consume at least 60% alkaline-producing foods in our diet, in order to maintain health. A healthy diet is one containing plenty of fresh fruits and particularly vegetables (alkaline-producing) to balance our necessary protein intake (acid-producing). You need to avoid processed, sugary or simple-carbohydrate foods, not only because they are acid-producing but also because they raise blood sugar levels too quickly - with high glycaemic index, therefore fattening and stressing our insulin response - plus they tend to be nutrient-lacking.

The body maintains the correct pH in the blood at all costs, by homeostasis, but that is stressful for the body's systems and resources when the diet is unbalanced in terms of acid-forming foods. When the pH in the blood becomes acidic, toxins are downloaded to every cell and organ in the body to adjust the blood pH balance in the blood. This mechanism makes all our organs act as a storehouse, by helping remove excess acidic toxins from the circulation, making our whole body acidic and toxic. High level of toxicity in the body cells is lethal; therefore the body's natural response is to dilute this toxicity with water retention. This is one of the reasons why people put on weight, not necessarily due to a high level of fat, but due to high level of water retention to dilute the body toxins. Saliva and urine tests show clearly the changes in alkalinity or acidity that are caused by

Emotional Detox Through Bodywork diet and lifestyle. No price can be placed on your health and research has shown that disease cannot exist in an alkaline state.

Why is the body's pH important?

An imbalanced diet high in acidic-producing foods such as meat, sugar, caffeine, and processed foods puts pressure on the body's regulating systems to maintain pH neutrality, depleting the body of alkaline minerals such as sodium, potassium, magnesium, and calcium, making the system susceptible to chronic and degenerative disease. Minerals are borrowed from vital organs and bones to neutralize the acid and safely remove it from the body. Because of this strain, the body can suffer severe and prolonged damage, a condition that may go undetected for years.

Health problems caused by acidosis

Research shows that unless the body's pH level is slightly alkaline, the body is unable to heal itself. So no matter how many gym memberships you hold, none of it will be effective until the pH level in your body is balanced. For example, if your body's pH is not balanced you cannot effectively assimilate vitamins, minerals and food supplements.

Acidosis causes the following health issues:

Decreases the body's ability to absorb minerals and other nutrients,
Decreases the energy production in the cells,
Decreases the body's ability to repair damaged cells, Decreases the body's ability to detoxify heavy metals,
Makes cancerous cells thrive,
Makes the body more susceptible to fatigue and illness.

An acidic pH can occur from an acid-forming diet, emotional stress, toxic overload, immune reactions or any process that deprives the cells of oxygen and other nutrients. The body will try to compensate for acidic pH by using alkaline minerals, thus deleting the body's natural reserves, however, if the diet does not contain enough minerals to compensate, a build-up of acids in the cells will occur.

Acidosis can cause such problems that include:

Cardiovascular damage. Weight gain, obesity and diabetes. Bladder conditions. Kidney stones. Immune deficiency. Acceleration of free radical damage. Hormonal problems. Premature aging. Osteoporosis and joint pain. Aching muscles and lactic acid build-up. Low energy and chronic fatigue.

Slow digestion and elimination. Yeast/fungal overgrowth. Lack of energy and fatigue. Lower body temperature. Tendency to get infections. Loss of drive, joy, and enthusiasm. Depressive tendencies. Easily stressed. Pale complexion. Headaches. Inflammation of the corneas and eyelids.

Loose and painful teeth. Inflamed, sensitive gums. Mouth and stomach ulcers. Cracks at the corners of the lips. Excess stomach acid. Gastritis. Nails are thin and split easily. Hair looks dull, has split ends, and falls out. Dry skin. Skin easily irritated. Leg cramps and spasms.

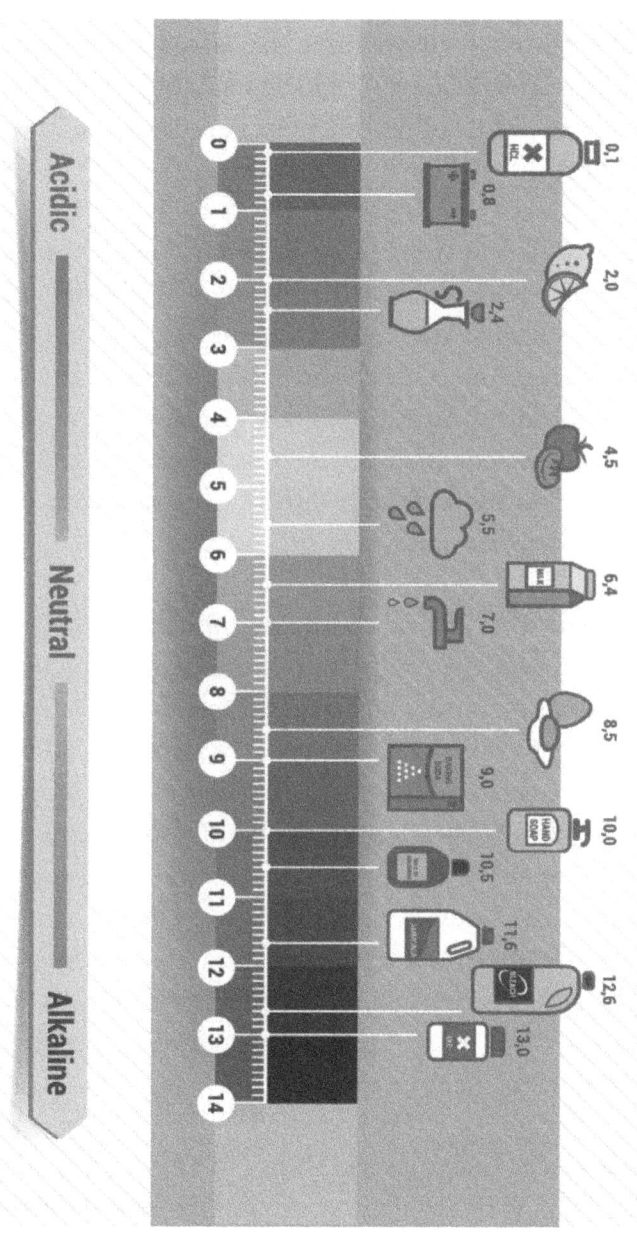

Test Your Body's Acidity or Alkalinity with pH Strips

It is recommended that you test your pH levels to determine if your body's pH needs immediate attention. By using pH test strips (Litmus Paper), you can determine your pH level quickly and easily. The best time to test your pH is either one hour before a meal and then two hours after a meal.

Saliva pH Test: Simply wet a piece of Litmus Paper with your saliva. While generally more acidic than blood, salivary pH mirrors the blood and tells us what the body retains. It is a fair indicator of the health of the extracellular fluids and their alkaline mineral reserves. The optimal pH for saliva is 6.4 to 6.8. A reading lower than 6.4 is indicative of insufficient alkaline reserves. After eating, the saliva pH should rise to 7.5 or more. If your saliva stays between 6.5 and 7.5 all day, your body is functioning within a healthy range.

Urine pH Test: The pH of the urine indicates how the body is working to maintain the proper pH of the blood. The urine reveals the alkaline (anabolic) and acid (catabolic) metabolic cycles. The pH of urine indicates the efforts of the body via the kidneys, adrenals, lungs and gonads to regulate pH through the reserve salts and hormones. Urine can provide a fairly accurate picture of body chemistry, because the kidneys filter out the salts of pH regulation and provide values based on what the body is eliminating. Urine pH can vary from around 4.5 to 9.0 in extremes, but the ideal range is 6.0 to 7.0. If your urinary pH fluctuates between 6.0 to 6.5 first thing in the morning and between 6.5 and 7.0 in the evening before dinner, your body is functioning within a healthy range.

The pH level of the body has the ability to affect every single cell of the body and the primary goal of an alkaline diet is usually to eat approximately 75-80% alkaline foods along with only about 20-25% acidifying foods. If this level is maintained in the diet a slightly alkaline pH in the body should be achieved.

Foods for an Alkaline Diet

It's actually quite easy to eat a diet rich in alkaline-producing foods. Most fresh fruits and vegetables are excellent choices. Red meat is not a good choice, but you can add plenty of protein to your meals by using soy products, delicious beans, legumes, and nuts such as almonds.

Use the food charts below to make your lifestyle more alkaline and reap the benefits of vibrant health and abundant energy...

FOOD CATEGORY	High Alkaline	Alkaline	Low Alkaline	Low Acid	Acid	High Acid
BEANS, VEGETABLES, PULSES	Vegetable Juices, Parsley, Raw Spinach, Broccoli, Celery, Garlic	Carrots, Green Beans, Beets, Lettuce, Butter Beans, Courgette	Squash, Asparagus, Rhubarb, Fresh Corn, Mushrooms, Onions, Cabbage, Peas, Cauliflower, Turnip, Beetroot, Potato, Olives, Soybeans, Tofu	Sweet Potato, Cooked Spinach, Kidney Beans	Pinto Beans, Haricot Beans	Pickled Vegetables
FRUIT	Dried Figs, Raisins	Dates, Blackcurrant, Grapes, Papaya, Kiwi, Berries, Apples, Pears	Coconut, Sour Cherries, Tomato's, Oranges, Cherries, Pineapple, Peaches, Avocados, Grapefruit, Mangoes, Strawberries, Papayas, Lemons, Watermelon, Limes	Blueberries, Cranberries, Bananas, Plums, Processed Fruit Juices	Canned Fruit	
GRAINS, CEREALS			Amaranth, Lentils, Sweetcorn, Wild Rice, Quinoa, Millet, Buckwheat	Rye Bread, Whole Grain Bread, Oats, Brown Rice	White Rice, White Bread, Pastries, Biscuits, Pasta	

MEAT				Liver, Oysters, Organ Meat	Fish, Turkey, Chicken, Lamb	Beef, Pork, Veal, Shellfish, Canned Tuna & Sardines
EGGS & DAIRY		Breast Milk	Soy Cheese, Soy Milk, Goat Milk, Goat Cheese, Buttermilk, Whey	Whole Milk, Butter, Yogurt, Cottage Cheese, Cream, Ice Cream	Eggs, Camembert, Hard Cheese	Parmesan, Processed Cheese
NUTS & SEEDS		Hazelnuts, Almonds	Chestnuts, Brazils, Coconut	Pumpkin, Sesame, Sunflower Seeds	Pecans, Cashews, Pistachios	Peanuts, Walnuts
OILS			Flax Seed Oil, Olive Oil	Corn Oil, Sunflower Oil, Margarine, Lard		
BEVERAGES	Herb Teas, Lemon Water	Green Tea	Ginger Tea	Cocoa	Wine, Soda/Pop	Tea (black), Coffee, Beer, Liquors
SWEETENERS, CONDIMENTS	Stevia (Stevia is a sweetener and sugar substitute extracted from the leaves of the plant species Stevia rebaudiana)	Maple Syrup, Rice Syrup	Raw Honey, Raw Sugar	White Sugar, Processed Honey	Milk Chocolate, Brown Sugar, Molasses, Jam, Ketchup, Mayonnaise, Mustard, Vinegar	Artificial Sweeteners

Following this chart will make planning balanced acid-alkaline meals easy

Foods: are they Acid or Alkaline-forming?

It is important to note that a food's acid or alkaline-forming tendency in the body has nothing to do with the actual pH of the food itself. For example, lemons are very acidic; however the end-products they produce after digestion and assimilation are alkaline so lemons are alkaline-forming in the body. Likewise, meat will test alkaline before digestion but it leaves acidic residue in the body so, like nearly all animal derived products, meat is classified as acid-forming.

The principles are clear: eat plenty of vegetables, some fruit daily, and don't eat *too much* of dairy products, grain products, and direct protein from eggs, meat and fish (as is typically the case in Western diet). This doesn't mean that you must abstain from all the meals that you enjoy, but instead by being conscious of the acidic value of ingredients in your diet you can shift your system towards an alkaline one.

Detoxify with Fruit & Vegetable Juices

All natural, raw, vegetable and fruit juices are alkaline-producing. (Fruit juices become more acid-producing when processed and sweetened so try to avoid shop purchased juices unless they are natural and freshly prepared).

A simple Alkaline Detox Juice Recipe

7 leaves Kale
1 large handful of fresh Basil
1 Cucumber
2 bulbs of Fennel
4 large Carrots
1 inch of raw Ginger root

Place all the ingredients into a juicer or liquidiser. This juice is alkalizing and is a good addition to an alkaline diet.

What are female sexual difficulties?

As I've indicated earlier within the introduction of this book, all of my clients are women. This is because it helps us to preserve the yin-yang balance as my female clients need the healing to be brought forth by a man in order to experience emotional release. There's also something to be said about how and why women are more often emotionally traumatized than men.

Contrary to popular belief, the female population is not the only sufferers of sexual dysfunction. The majority of people are aware of erectile dysfunction, impotence and issues that relate to male sexuality; however, it is estimated that four out of ten British women suffer from sexual dysfunction. Despite it being common it is still largely ignored. There are still are a lot of myths associated with the sexuality of women and a lot is still not understood in mainstream Western medicine. Sexual dysfunction is defined as an inability to experience pleasure during intercourse. For main stream medical professionals most women's sexual problems are not a priority or cause for concern, but for the women who experience sexual difficulties it can lead to depression, guilt, and feelings of isolation, the breakdown of relationships and negative body image.

Couples suffering with "Unhappy Marriages"

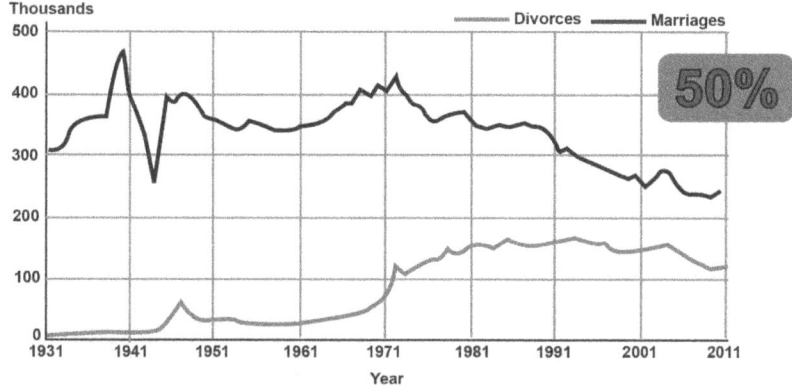

Divorce and marriage in England and Wales

Statistics on women's orgasm;
- 12% anorgasmic(never had an orgasm)
- 75% Can't have an orgasm through sex
- 85% Can't ejaculate
- 40% Suffer sexual dysfunctions
- 10% Suffer with Veganism (can't have sex)

Mainstream medicine still struggles to diagnose and effectively treat female sexual dysfunction. The symptoms can include lack of sexual desire, an inability to enjoy sex, pain during intercourse, insufficient vaginal lubrication or, even if sexually aroused, a failure to achieve an orgasm leading to feelings of inadequacy, depression and alienation. According to The Sexual Advice Association, sexual problems affect around fifty per cent of women, making it a common problem that remains largely unheard of. Furthermore it is reported that eighty per cent of women who seek help for sexual dysfunction complain of having no sexual desire, libido, tiredness, depression, illness, stress, anxiety, relationship disharmony and negative body image, which means that this problem is extending into all areas of these women's lives.

Often women do not seek help through embarrassment or for fear of being labelled or fear of being inadequate. Those who do seek help often find that the treatment offered falls short of their needs and results in a deeper sense of despair. Talking about sexual dysfunction can become a great obstacle, which is why many couples choose to ignore it rather than face the awkwardness of discussion or for fear of abnormality. Indeed, it is only when relationships are at a breaking point that they finally search for help.

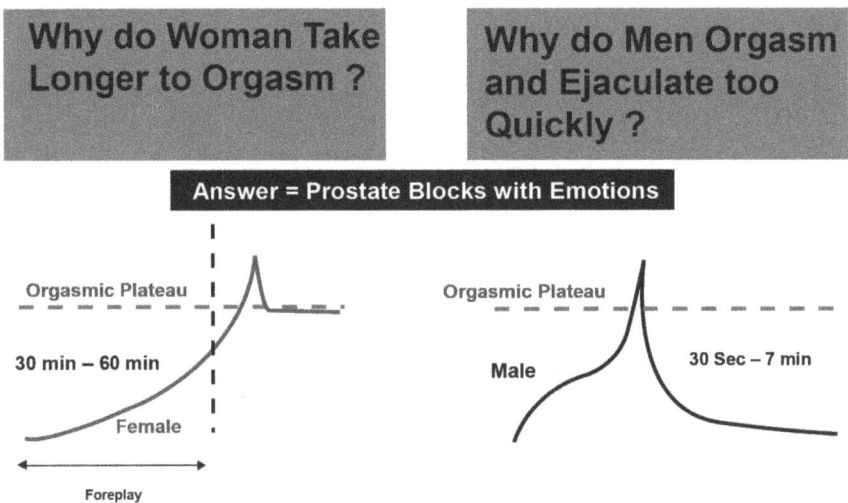

Fortunately, times appear to be changing and women desperate to improve their quality of life are beginning to take action and seek help. More women want to be in charge of their sexual lives, meaning they want to know why they find it difficult to be sexually satisfied by a partner or why they're suffering from sexual dysfunction.

Many women feel a deep need for transformation. Healing takes place by having a different experience and avoiding intimacy can keep you trapped. Traditional therapy focuses on working through pain and trauma; Tantric Journey offers the additional possibility that experiences of bliss can heal and dissolve held pain.

Many women are often unaware that they're suffering from sexual dysfunction, especially in today's popular society which highlights how men are always desperate for sex, and women should be sexual moral compasses.

However, you'd be surprised at how many people could consider themselves to be sexually dysfunctional and not know it.

Orgasmic wave of a Unhappy Woman.

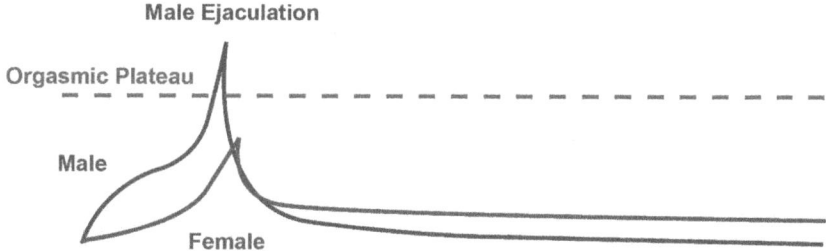

Dr. Wilhem Reich, the pioneer psychotherapist and sexologist who postulated the orgasm theory, proclaimed that full orgasm is the very center of human experience and ultimately determines the happiness of the human race

Consider asking yourself the following questions to see where you stand:

1. Have you ever felt incomplete during sex because your partner has already "landed" before you have even had a chance to "take off"?
2. Have you ever glimpsed an ecstatic moment in love and later felt that you did not know the way back?
3. Have you ever wished to be touched at the core of your being, yet felt afraid to open yourself up and be vulnerable?

4. Have you ever felt bored with sex in a long-term relationship and found yourself wishing you could capture the passion that used to make sex between you so exciting?

5. Whilst making love or just afterwards, have you ever wondered: Isn't there more to sex, than this?

6. Do you find it difficult to find a suitable lifelong partner or to maintain a satisfying long-term relationship?

If you identified with any of the above questions, it's likely that you suffer from some form of sexual dysfunction, whether it stems from emotional roots (i.e. past traumatic experiences or negative events) or physical ailments. However, now that you've answered these questions, ask yourself how likely it is that you'd seek out Tantric Journey to help you achieve a fulfilling sexual relationship.

If you're like most women, chances are you're not very likely to do so at all. It's easy to see why. The arena of sexual awakening can often be judged harshly by others as being shameful, dangerous or seedy. In my experience nothing could be further from the truth. It is a deeply spiritual treatment, which offers healing across a wide range of issues.

A client I treated early in my career found a reversal in the cancerous cells of the cervix following several treatments, and another who suffered from vaginismus (an involuntary closing of the vagina, making penetration impossible) was finally able to make love with her husband after 12 years. Most of my clients find either vast improvement in their intimate relationships, or that they are able to attract a successful partner into their life. Menstrual problems are frequently resolved, as are numerous sexual dysfunctions, including inability to or difficulty with orgasm, emotional issues, insomnia, depression and body aches and stresses.

At the heart of the treatment for the client is often the discovery of female ejaculation for the first time. The production and release of this amrita, as it is called, heralds a new level of vitality and relaxation, which is profoundly healing. However, so many women are afraid of achieving – even demanding – an orgasm in the same way that men often do. It's expected that men will orgasm; the female orgasm is seen as non-mandatory consequence.

That's why so many women benefit from the Tantric Journey, because they learn that the female orgasm is not something to be afraid of; rather, it's a pleasurable pursuit that can help them reach their highest potential.

My advanced techniques can help remove any negative roadblocks that cause female impotence. After all, you have the right to feel happy, healthy, and fully satisfied with your life and there should be absolutely no shame in seeking out emotional release through Bodywork as a means to reconnect yourself with your sexual essence.

The amount of power you have is enormous and Tantric Journey can open up your mind and body to that incredible power. The goal of my treatments and of the methods I describe within this book are to make you independent and not dependent. The female orgasm is a holistic experience involving a woman's mind, body and emotions; it is not dependent on the skills of her partner, as the key to orgasm is held by the woman herself.

What Is Tantra and Tao Practice?

Picture what Tantra is in your mind's eye, and you'll probably see a visualization of two people entwined with one another, enjoying a sexual marathon of bended poses and positions and night-long sex sessions. If this is exactly what you pictured, it's important to note that this doesn't accurately reflect Tantra; in fact, far from it.

Work in this field is largely misunderstood and for many, the misunderstanding is that, sexual arousal and fantastic sex are the main focus of Tantra. This misconception stems from the fact that Tantra accepts sexual energy and harnesses it as a route to higher consciousness. This has been largely misinterpreted in the West, as meaning Tantra merely focuses on achieving sexual ecstasy. It has subsequently gained a reputation of being outside the pale of respectability and in the minds of many it brands female Tantric healers as sex workers and male Tantric healers as sexual predators.

The fact that Tantra treats sexual energy as an ally, rather than something to be suppressed or hushed up makes many people feel uncomfortable within the concept of the therapy. This stems from lack of understanding. Tantric Journey work does not deny sexual energy; it embraces sexual energy, but that does not mean the same thing as sex which is how the unenlightened media defines it.

In the work I do sexual energy is used as ignition for firing the Kundalini energy, the body's biological energy system, merging it with universal energy. Indeed the work I do can help a person enjoy their sex life to its fullest potential, but it is far wider reaching than that. It can help to break down barriers of guilt or fear, and remove self-imposed or limiting cultural and social boundaries. It releases emotional pain which has been trapped within the body and allows the body's own responses to facilitate healing and balance.

The word Tantra is a Sanskrit word which means, to weave, to transform through methods, and to transform poison into nectar or negativity into positivity. This description of Tantra offers a far better insight into the true transformational nature of the discipline. My work is all about helping people to gain release from negative emotional trauma through Tantric Journey Bodywork and transform their lives, emerging like a butterfly from a chrysalis.

When entangled with unhappiness from the past, people often adopt patterns of anxiety, depression, anger, guilt, fear, chronic illness and unfulfilled relationships. This is because negative emotions as a result of trauma are not resolved; they physically embed as a cellular memory in the body cells, thus preventing these cells from playing their optimum part by constant biochemical entanglement and communication taking place within the body. These memories not only 'switch off' these cells, but lead to emotional and physical disease years after the events originally occurred. What Tantric Journey looks to achieve is the optimal flow of energy in the body that is renewable and expandable.

These time tested methodologies and beliefs have been well tested over thousands of years, not in worldly laboratories but in the laboratories of the human body, by Yogi Scientists and Tibetan Lamas who were not driven by commerce but by the earnest desire for spiritual knowledge and liberation. Their observations and insights have been passed down to us.

Tantric Journey is not a philosophy that requires a modern-day householder to renounce the world by giving up family, job, possessions, and pleasures. Instead, it emphasizes personal experimentation and experience as a way to move forward on the path to self-realization.

When undergoing Tantric Journey with my clients, I follow a three step treatment plan:

1. **Talking Therapy:** this opens the mind and allows clients to begin getting comfortable with me to develop connection and trust. It also allows clients to be vocal in their expectations for their sessions with me. It is through this process that I establish their aims, fears and boundaries. Talking therapy helps the client to accept and embark into Bodywork.

2. **Body Therapy:** this is where I use deep tissue massages to transform places of numbness into places of pleasure (through subtle pain), thus releasing emotional trauma that has been trapped at the cellular level. Deep Bodywork makes the client go into an altered state of consciousness (a trance state) making them receptive for deeper healing.

3. **Yoni Massage:** this allows the client to open the spirit through ejaculation, thus releasing negative emotions from the physical body.

This is often the point where Tantra receives its reputation, which is wholly unfair and subjected to multiple Western prejudices. This is why I want to take a moment to explain the concept of the yoni massage and how it can be incorporated into the Tantric Journey.

"Yoni" is the Sanskrit word for the vagina, which literally translates to "Divine Passage." Yoni massage is the ritual of honouring and healing this part of the body. In this ritual, you touch the yoni not from a place of arousal and orgasm, but from a joy and wonder of this beautiful part of the body with unconditional love and respect on a safe, sacred platform.

A woman's sexuality is located in her heart and mind; however, much of her trauma is held in her yoni. A yoni massage clears away this trauma through female ejaculation, which helps the woman open up to a new level of sexual experiences while giving the body emotional release. Yoni massage will often bring more sensitivity and aliveness to the female g-spot, and lead to the amazing experience of female ejaculation, which releases amrita, the sacred feminine waters.

Through this sacred ritual, you learn to release old beliefs that are keeping you from your full potential as a lover, and your full enjoyment of your sexuality. The goal of the yoni massage is not solely to achieve orgasms, although orgasms are often pleasant and welcome sign posts. The goal can be as simple as to fully feel the physical and emotional pain and to let go of these negative stagnant emotions and trauma from the body and to give permission for the yoni to feel deeper pleasure.

This process of healing the yoni is a lot like weeding a garden; you must pull the weeds out in order to allow the beautiful flowers to grow. Yoni massage is not a sexual treatment, but an emotional release treatment.

Ancient Practice, Modern Uses

No examination of the art of Tantra would be complete without first examining its history. According to Nik Douglas, a spiritual writer, the meaning of Tantra given in his book Spiritual Sex, "Tantra is a spiritual science, which means it is also mystical, in its interconnectedness, the holistic wisdom link between ourselves and the universe we inhabit".

"By embracing Tantra, we become more "real," more "complete." How? By recognizing and stimulating our inherent sensual spirituality, we discover parts of ourselves that have remained asleep or have been repressed. With Tantra, an energy is released that is evolutionary and "upwardly motivated." We can learn to use this energy for pleasure, for achieving our worldly goals, and for aiding our spiritual evolution".

"Familiarity with Tantra can help a person to enjoy life to the fullest. It can help do away with guilt or fear, break down self-imposed or limiting cultural boundaries, and guide us in our search for solutions. Tantra teaches us to become familiar with our mystical nature, and when we do so, our boundaries expand. We enter into new domains of awareness. We become empowered, more fulfilled, and more perfect".

"Traditional dictionary definitions of Tantra are revealing. A Sanskrit word, Tantra is sometimes translated as "leading principle, essential part, model, system, framework, doctrine, rule, theory, scientific mystic works, magical formulas, means, expedient, stratagem, medicine." Finally, a Tantra is sometimes defined as "a type of mystical teaching set out mostly in the form of dialogs between a cosmic couple. Intimate insightful dialogs, between God and Goddess, Shiva and Shakti, the male and female Tantric adepts, were at times written down and became known as Tantras. Naturally, these dialogs, being intimate, included sexual secrets as well as many other fascinating topics".

"The sacred Hindu and Buddhist scriptures known as Tantras provide detailed instructions on a wide range of topics, including spiritual knowledge, technology, and science. Their content is often paradoxical. In Tantra, science and mysticism go hand in hand, as do sensuality and asceticism. Just as advanced scientific treatises are difficult for the layperson to comprehend, so traditional Tantras require adequate preparation before they can be properly understood".

Tantra started 5,000 years ago in India. From India it went to China and they called it Tao. All of this spiritual work which was empowering women actually happened in the Asian countries; in the Far East. Women were treated equally and even during Buddha's time Buddha said that women are as equal as men. Women were allowed to come to partake in the religion and to meet priests and so forth.

Whilst India had a wealth of knowledge and a rich heritage, much of the true meaning and teachings of Tantra have been lost due to the foreign onslaught over the past millennium and for reasons of selfish endeavour and ignorance, Tantra's reputation has been sullied.

History of female ejaculation

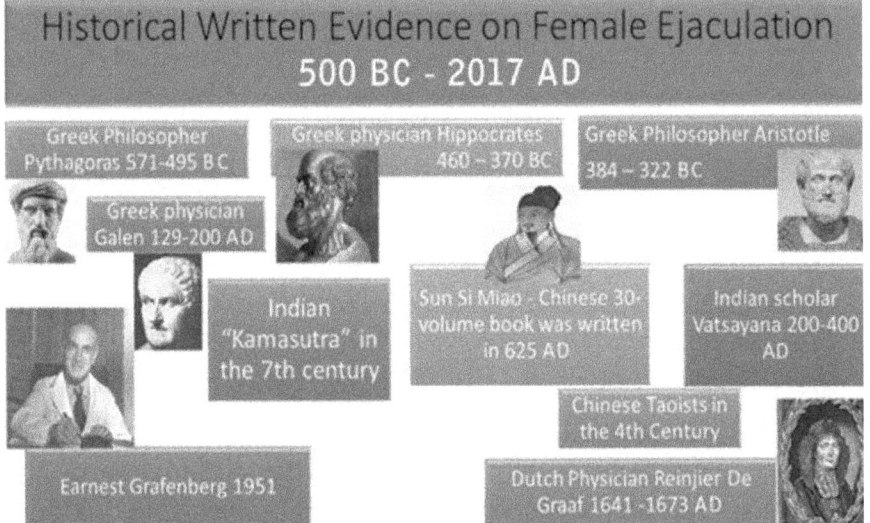

Historical Written Evidence on Female Ejaculation 500 BC - 2017 AD

Greek Philosopher Pythagoras 571-495 B C

Greek physician Galen 129-200 AD

Greek physician Hippocrates 460 – 370 BC

Greek Philosopher Aristotle 384 – 322 BC

Indian "Kamasutra" in the 7th century

Sun Si Miao - Chinese 30-volume book was written in 625 AD

Indian scholar Vatsayana 200-400 AD

Chinese Taoists in the 4th Century

Earnest Grafenberg 1951

Dutch Physician Reinjier De Graaf 1641 -1673 AD

The study of ejaculation has been evidently recorded throughout the early years by many physicians and anatomists in books, poems, and research papers. The earliest writings being recorded are by Aristotle in 300 BC, to the Chinese Taoists in the 4th Century in the classical text "Secret Instructions in the Jade Chamber", mentioned in a 7th century Indian poem where detailed description is given in the "Kamasutra" and in an article in 1951 called "The role of the urethra in female ejaculation" by Earnest Grafenberg.

Nick Fleming in 2006 writes that "the phenomenon of female ejaculation and the female prostate is not the construct of modern society. Historical references of female ejaculation begin over 2000 years ago with Aristotle who noted that some women expelled a fluid during orgasm." *[A Review of Female Ejaculation During Orgasm by Nick Fleming]*

The ancient Chinese, who believed sexual intercourse to be the foundation of life, perceived ejaculation in a philosophical manner using the concept of Yin and Yang -- Yin being female and Yang male. A woman's Yin essence was believed to be of negative energy and evil of inexhaustible supply and a man's Yang superior, pure and positive but of a limited supply. As a preventive measure, a man was advised to prolong his ejaculation and to orgasm the woman many times to acquire her Yin essence, thus avoiding health problems and even possibly death. A man capable of making a woman ejaculate is believed to be healthy and will have longevity.

Deborah Sundah in 'Female Ejaculation and the G-spot', stated that the "knowledge of female ejaculation is by no means new. Cultures around the world have left records showing that they knew of its existence, and viewed it as natural, normal, and, in some cases, healing and sacred. The openness of some of these cultures towards female ejaculation illustrates how modern Western society is actually unusual in its ignorance about these feminine 'flow waters'.

China

Talltrees and Pokras say, "Ancient Chinese texts make reference to a woman's water flowing".

A Chinese classic 30-volume book was written in 625 AD by Sun Si Miao called "Prescriptions Worth a Thousand Pieces of Gold". In a chapter of this Taoist text, it is quoted, "If for example, the male is not yet excited you must wait till he becomes agitated. Therefore, control your feelings somewhat so as to respond in concert with him.

In any event, you must not shake and dance about, causing your female fluid to be exhausted first". The author uses the term "female fluid" which can be interpreted as female ejaculation. The possibility of the "female fluid" being pernicious can be removed as the author does not talk about the Yin essence which is being earlier mentioned as evidently inexhaustible.

India

A Seventh century poem, called "Amarushataka" written by Amaru, a king and warlord, is believed to be oldest piece of literature on female ejaculation found in Indian history. A German Indologist called Syed, interpreted the term "love juice" as female ejaculate. The following is the poem:

Her breasts were compressed in close embracement,
Frisson of excitement apprehended her torso,
Smooth love juice overflowed abundantly the garment,
Right there where her girdle was located;
"Don't! Don't! Wrecker of my pride, back off, this is
Enough for me"
So she moaned, to obtain mercy.
Did she sleep, did she
Die then?
Sink into my heart
["Amarushataka", stave 35]

In 200 – 400 AD the Kamasutra was written in the Sanskrit language and describes the permissible goals of life. This has over the centuries become misunderstood and interpreted as a sex manual full of exploratory love making positions. However, despite misconceptions held by some, it is still considered the primary Sanskrit work on human sexuality. According to tradition, the companion of Shiva, Nandi, overheard the god making love to his wife Parvati and was consequently inspired, thus leading to the writing of the original Kama Sutra. It is then told that the scholar Vatsayana redacted this version between 200-400 AD. It is a very important text as it records ancient Indian practices and knowledge. The male and female semen are evidently mentioned within its pages. In one passage it reads, "The fall of the semen of the man takes place only at the end of coition, while the semen of the woman falls continually, and after the semen of both has all fallen away then the wish for discontinuance of coition". The "female semen" referred to here is evidently the female ejaculation.

The Ratirahasya (translated in English as the Secrets of Love, also known as the Koka Shastra) is a medieval Indian manual of love, written by Kokkoka, a poet, who is variously described as Koka or Koka Pundit. The exact date of its writing is not known, but it is estimated the text was written in the Eleventh or Twelfth century.

In 12th Century AD the poet Kukkoka, wrote "Ratirahasiya", the earliest work after Kamasutra. As translated by Syed, the vagina contains many veins of "love water". It described an itching ("kanduti") which can be eliminated by vigorous rubbing of the man's penis ("candadhvaja") or (hot bar), consequently creating the flow of the vagina fluid ("ksarana"), which is followed by an orgasm ('sukha"). As quoted in this text, "The woman who has emitted the water of the one whose arrow is of flowers at the end of coitus dances with much jumping and crying". "Water" being female ejaculate and taking into consideration it is mentioned upon emission of the "water" a woman jumps and cries which we can relate to a pleasurable orgasm through emotional release, hence validating the fact Kukkoka was describing female ejaculation in his poem.

Das further translates work of another author, Yasodhara who wrote "Jayamangala" in 1300 AD. Yasodhara describes female ejaculation and provides evidence through comparing the time of the male and female ejaculation, which distinguishes lubrication during foreplay and ejaculation. He states," That both male and female experience the delight of emission (visrsti-), the woman, however, from the beginning of intercourse, for she gradually becomes, as can be perceived, wet like a broken water vessel. Her delight is conjoined with an emission (visrsti-) like that of the man, accompanied by bhava-, from the beginning, while the man's bhava- is obtained at the end, because of the voiding (visarga-) of semen (sukra-). Their delight of emission (visrsti-) is the same, though not the time".

Western Ancient World

Female ejaculation was mentioned by ancient Greek philosophers Pythogoras (570-510 BC) and Empedocles (490 – 430 BC) in reproductive texts. "Father of Medicine" Hippocrates had a more controversial viewpoint on female ejaculation and even believed it necessary for conception. He further believed the sex of the child was determined by the strength and volume of emission of the ejaculation. He states 'On Generation', "A woman also emits something from her body, sometimes into the womb, which then becomes moist, and some- times externally as well . . . If her desire for intercourse is excited, she emits before the man". He doesn't give a specific terminology for female ejaculation but evidently states that there is external expulsion of fluid. Which comes out externally from G-spot stimulation and the internal ejaculation comes from A-spot stimulation.

Aristotle in (384 – 322 BC) describes in the "On the Generation of Animals", that there is a discharge from the uterus and the amount of discharge varies and in some cases it is larger than male semen. He says, "The female also projects her semen into the os uteri, where the man also emits his . . . There is a tube enclosed in the body like the penis of the male . . . When therefore they desire sexual intercourse, this part is not in the same condition as it was before . . . Whatever conjecture is formed concerning these affections, it makes to the same conclusion, that woman also emits a seminal fluid".

Claudius Galenus of Pergamum (129-200 AD), the last doctor of antiquity, is the first to provide evidence on female ejaculation on non-sex basis but through anatomical observation. He dispersed the doctrine that woman's reproductive system is an overturned version of a man's genitals. Following is textual exemplification on the evident female ejaculation expulsed during sexual pleasure, 'In the case of a woman suffering from hysterical diseases, very abundant and very thick semen was discharged first to the uterus and from it to the outside; a widow for a long time, she had collected it in that amount and of that kind. But then certain tensions seized her in her loins and hands and feet, so that she seemed convulsed ('spasthenai'), and at these tensions the semen was discharged ('ex-ekrithe'), and she said that the pleasure it gave her was like that of sexual intercourse". The convulsion observed occurs to disperse the stuck negative energy held within the body and to ejaculate is to further eliminate stuck negative energy resulting in the experience of a deep orgasm.

He concluded women like men needed to release their induced – accumulated pain and the Galenic egalitarian homology spread through the empire of Persia.

The first strictly scientific insight on female ejaculation was done by Reinjier De Graaf (1641-1673 AD). He gave a morphological description of the female reproductive system and provided the first literature on the anatomy of female ejaculation and coined the term, "female prostate". He effectively differentiates female ejaculate from the male semen and identifies its source of production and highlights the fact it is produced by pleasure during coitus. The following text is an anatomical description of the glands responsible to produce the ejaculate, "There will doubtless be critics who, believing that the liquid which rushes out with such impetus during veneral combat or libidinous imaging is semen, will enquire whence this liquid comes and for what purpose it is designed. We think that it comes primarily from the lacunae in the orifices of the vagina and the urinary tract . . . The first-mentioned ducts, namely those which are visible around the orifice of the neck of the vagina and the outlet of the urinary passage receive their fluid from the female parastatae, or rather the thick membranous body around the urinary passage"

Germany

In 1951, Dr Earnest Grafenberg states in his paper, "The role of the urethra in female ejaculation" that "occasionally the production of fluids is so profuse that a large towel has to be spread under the woman to prevent the bed sheets getting soiled. This convulsory expulsion of fluids occurs always at the acme of the orgasm and simultaneously with it". And he further states, "At first I thought that the bladder sphincter had become defective by the intensity of the orgasm. Involuntary expulsion of urine is reported in sex literature. In the cases observed by us, the fluid was examined and it had no urinary character. I am inclined to believe that "urine" reported to be expelled during female orgasm is not urine, but only secretions of the intraurethral glands correlated with the erotogenic zone along the urethra in the anterior vaginal wall." The above extracts from Granfenberg's report rules out all possibility that the secretion during the acme of an orgasm is urine or incontinence. And indeed women have been ejaculating on sexual stimulation for many centuries.

Dr Earnst Granfenberg was a decorated individual who published at least twelve papers and a scientific researcher of importance. In 1940 he left Germany after his arrest during the war and upon arrival in America he worked as a Pathologist in Chicago and later moved to New York City.

After the terming of the female prostrate by Reinjier De Graaf, Grafenberg provided a breakthrough in understanding the functional anatomy of female sexual organs.

Other Terms Used For Female Ejaculation

- Amrita – ancient Tantric text
- Divine Nectar – ancient Tantric text
- "Liquid of energy" by Caroline Muir, Founder of Divine Feminine
- "Copious emissions" in the Secret Methods of the Plain Girl by Su Nu Ching in 618 AD
- "Love water" by Kukkoka in Ratirahasiya
- "Semen of the woman" by Mallanaga in Kamasutra
- "Love juice" by Amaru in Amarushataka
- "Kama salila" by the poet Kalyanamalla in his four orders of women
- "Passion water" by Revanaradhya in Samaratattvaprakasika
- "Seminal fluid" by Aristotle in On the Generation of Animals
- "Serous fluid' by Reinjier De Graaf, the first scientist who used the term "female prostate"
- "flowing water" by Deborah Sundahl
- "ambrosia" by Fulbright author of Touch Me
- "Yoni Crying" by Mal Weeraratne, Founder of Tantric Journey School of Healing and Awakening

There: A Hands-On Guide to Your Orgasmic Hot Spots!

Yvonne K. Fulbright further states that "because of its respected role in female ejaculation, tantric practitioners, refer to the G-spot as the 'sacred castle' or 'sacred spot'". With so much compelling evidence mentioning female ejaculation over the course of history, perhaps it's easy to see why the modern controversy over female ejaculation and the G-spot today can be considered somewhat ludicrous. We'll discuss female ejaculation in a later chapter of this book.

Tantric Bodywork to Evoke Negative Imprints

I often refer to a Tantric Journey treatment as awakening of the female energy, and it is undertaken gradually, with respect for each individual, primarily by helping them to evoke and release their stagnant negative emotions, energies, thoughts, feelings, actions and beliefs. Women are primarily emotional bodies, in contrast to men who are primarily logical bodies. Emotions can be both positively charged or negatively charged. Women's emotional network connection in the body is far sharper than a man's and deeply connected to the sex centre both due to a protective mechanism as a result of their negative emotions such as fear, shame etc. In the same manner due to this complex emotional link, once the negative emotions are removed from the body, they are able to connect any part of their body with the sex centre through the positive emotional network. This is an amazing gift women have. This means that women can experience joy and ecstasy through any part of their body more easily than men, whose energy is more focused genitally. Men lack such bodily connections due to their logical mind and have reduced emotional connections in comparison to women. Men's sex is in the mind at all times and mostly stimulated only via direct genital stimulation rather than other body parts.

However, it also means that a woman is more likely to shut down a part of her body due to negative emotions as a result of trauma and stress. When we absorb negative emotions, the first thing that happens is that they are buried in our cells, causing pain which eventually becomes so chronic we shut off our perception and experience numbness. Women, being emotional in their bodies, do this more frequently than men.

Breathing is incredibly important to the Tantric Journey process because it helps us to release toxins from our bodies. There are two types of toxins that are removed from the body during these breathing exercises: physical toxins, and emotional toxins. Breathing helps to release evoked emotions, which helps an individual bring repressed feelings and memories to the surface.

How do Organs get Blocked?

Blocked Capillaries

1. Sedimentation as a result of Physical Toxins due to what we Eat, Drink, Breath (Smoke)

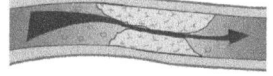

Knots & Tangles Formation

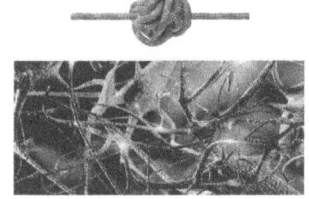

2. Knots and Tangles as a result of Emotional Toxins due to Stress & Trauma

Breathing and emotions are inextricably tied together. Think of the small child who is angry or upset, and wants to avoid showing these feelings. Chances are that he or she will hold his or her breath until he or she begins feeling better. This is a natural instinct within humans, as our bodies impulsively tell us to hold our breath when a strong emotion is threatening to take over. It is natural to retain breath for fear of fully feeling the emotions. If we fully feel the emotion and breathe into it, we let go of the very emotion.

Think about a time when you were running so fast that you felt out of breath. When you were trying to catch your breath, your body felt like it was in pain. But as you took big gulps of air, your body slowly started to feel normal again. This is similar to what happens during Tantric Journey Bodywork, as deep breaths can help my clients experience the kind of healing that will make them feel "normal" again.

During Bodywork, I ensure that my clients are breathing in through the nose, and out through the mouth (I refer to this as "Tantric breathing"). What's more, I remind my clients to remain conscious of their breathing throughout this process. I tell them to repeat the phrase, "in through the nose, out through the mouth" until they're wholly focused on their breathing this practice focuses the mind and helps to eliminate mind chatter and thoughts drifting.

Deep breathing is critical for a successful session – after all, you have to get rid of negative emotions in order to make room for the positive ones that you will soon experience. Only when this focused level of breathing has been achieved can we engage in the kind of Bodywork that helps release emotional memories from the cellular level.

After we've achieved the focused breathing that's essential for Tantric Journey Bodywork, we'll use body movements to help spread positive energy throughout the entire physical self. To help illustrate the power of this, think of when you stroke a cat. When you reach down to stroke a cat, the cat gets its whole body involved in the enjoyable process. The cat's purring at full volume, its back arches to meet your hand, and its tail is twitching in delight. This is akin to what happens during Tantric Journey Bodywork, as physical movements can help keep the body flexible, which is essential for spreading positive emotions throughout the body.

During Bodywork, there's no specific way you need to move; the point is just to move. Do what feels natural to you, all while staying focused on your breathing. Give your body permission to feel pleasure, as this is essential for releasing negative emotions and making room for pleasure within the physical self.

Finally, I encourage my clients to make any noises that they want to express during Bodywork. There's no right or wrong way to express a noise, breathing or moving the body; just do what feels natural to you.

Releasing negative energy through vocalization can be essential to the healing process, as it allows you to verbally express the pain or pleasure you're feeling. This allows the positive energy you're experiencing to move past the throat by pulling the energy from the pelvic, upwards towards the crown, which is why it's so important to make sounds during the Bodywork process. Just as we don't want the body to be rigid, we don't want the vocal cords to be rigid either. The throat harbours many suppressed emotions that build up due to the inability to effectively express during trauma. To break down this rigidity it's important to release both positive and negative emotions verbally. Express your sadness and anger verbally as you release negative emotions as well as when you are in orgasmic ecstasy when you process positive emotions.

The Five Gateways

Intimacy plays a critical role in ensuring that a person is happy, healthy, and satisfied. Usually my clients have a problem with intimacy, more than sex or love. They may be capable of having sex, or feeling like they're in love, but they can never really achieve the true intimacy they're looking for because they haven't been able to release the negative emotions that are residing within them at the cellular level.

Intimacy can be represented by so many different emotions, which is why it's so critical for individuals to work on their intimacy issues if they want to learn how to have a fulfilling love life.

In general, intimacy is represented by five different senses, or gateways. Each gateway has two different points of entry and exit; therefore, because there are five gateways, we have ten ways in and out.

Now when somebody is traumatised at any stage, this trauma must happen through one of these gateways. It cannot happen any other way; they have seen something happening to somebody or heard, tasted, smelled or felt something happening. If the trauma enters through one of these gateways, Tantric Journey Bodywork can help it leave through the same gateway; this is why certain tantric rituals are so important, as they help to challenge the client in a safe and sacred environment. Such practices evoke the trauma related to intimacy and help to release emotions through breath and eye contact as well as empowering the client and aiding them in letting go of stuck emotions, an element that is so important to the healing process.

Let's examine the five gateways to learn why they're so critical to the Tantric Journey healing process.

Sight

Much of human communication is done through visual cues, which is why it's so important for clients to heighten their sense of intimacy through the sense of sight. To see if this gateway is blocked, I'll usually have a client look me in the eyes for a prolonged period of time. If the client begins to experience a level of discomfort, this usually means there has been some trauma that hasn't been resolved yet.

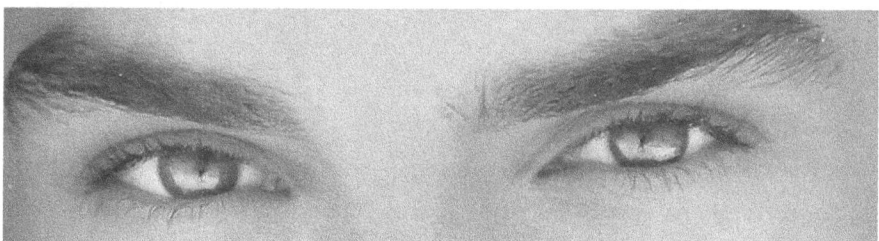

In order to heal this gateway, I'll have the client look me in the eyes throughout the breathing exercise until she's healed. Looking in the eyes of another can evoke a great deal of emotions, which is why it's so important to keep breathing so as to release these emotions.

When this gateway has been cleared, a client will find that it's easier for her to look her loved one in the eye, as she's no longer afraid or uncomfortable with this level of intimacy. When the sense of vision is open, it's possible to establish a deeper connection with each other at soul level.

Touch

Touch plays an important role in the healing process, as it teaches the client that touching can be a sensuous and pleasurable action. When I mention touch in this text, it simply means a gentle stroke of a person's body. To help understand what this means, put on a blindfold with a partner and pretend as though you're both two blind people who are meeting each other for the first time. The kind of touching you'd need to use in order to "see" each other will be very gentle yet knowledgeable; there's no sensuality or sexuality behind it. See if you can touch with consciousness like two blind people to get to know each other's size, explore different parts of the body, the texture of the skin and hair etc. Take time and notice so that if you met up many months later, amongst many hundreds of people, you would still be able to recognise and connect with each other just through touch. To do this exercise you need to shut off all other senses and focus on touch. Because we have vision we don't use touch as a way of connecting with people.

With some practice you will increase the awareness to touch and be more sensitive for both giving and receiving touch. If you have experienced trauma through touch in the past you would probably shut down this sense and become numb or feel uncomfortable to touch or to be touched this way.

This is how you evoke emotions and feel the discomfort which you need to fully feel in your whole body and breath into this emotion a few times until it goes away. After a few minutes you will feel the discomfort leave your body and you will feel pleasure. Then focus on the pleasure and give yourself permission to fully feel this pleasure and move on to another body part to find another challenging part of the body and do the same.

If this gateway is blocked up, the person will usually have a hard time engaging in this type of touching. The Tantric Journey healing process will clear up this blocked gateway by using this form of touching, which will help the person connect to a positive and loving experience.

Sound

Many people find it difficult to communicate with one another because there are a variety of emotions, sensations, beliefs, and values that are influencing how we all interpret one another. However, communication can become traumatic when it is used to cut another person down. For example, a client who grew up hearing that she was ugly or fat all the time is likely to have a traumatic block in this gateway, as she won't know how to communicate with another man unless it's being done in a negative and destructive manner.

To eliminate the negativity from this gateway, I work with the client to understand what she really wants to hear from the person she's intimate with, or what she wants from her communications with other people. Once we've established what she wants to hear, we begin to incorporate these positive mantras or affirmations into her breathing exercises. This can evoke emotions in a very subtle way, so that these negative feelings are breathed out of the body. For example you keep whispering in her ears that she is so beautiful, she is so sexy, and she has a slim body etc. and then get her to affirm the same: I am so beautiful, I am sexy, and I have a slim body. With these affirmations incorporating consciousness and breath, you heal the body that is connected to negative emotions through sounds.

What's funny is that this exercise can help my clients understand that they don't always need to hear what they want to hear from other people. They don't need people telling them that they're beautiful all the time, because this exercise can help them inherently see and believe in their own beauty. By removing the negativity from the gateway, I can help the client learn how to effectively communicate, which solves about 50% of their issues in the first place.

Dialogue is critical for connecting with another human being. Without this dialogue, it becomes difficult to establish intimacy with someone else. Tantric Journey can help bring these communication skills to life, thus helping my clients learn how to establish healthy relationships again. By being able to ask for exactly what they want, express how they want something and when they want something, they learn to communicate and strengthen their relationships. Similarly you learn how to say "No", or express what you don't like and don't want. This ability could become very empowering to a woman who has been in silence all her life without knowing how to speak her own truth.

Now in relation to how sound moves through the body; energy moves upwards from the pelvis towards the head, through the body. If you have a look at our body, you will see we have our body's trunk. It is wider at the bottom and then when it comes up to the neck, it squeezes and gets thin, like a bottle neck. Our head sits upon the thin neck. Imagine, if you will, the powerful energy from the pelvic area moving upwards through the body and attempting to exit through the top of your head at the Crown Chakra.

This orgasmic sexual energy travels in waves within the body, all pushing upwards towards the crown. Of course, as it comes closer to our neck, it becomes cramped, crushed even. Much like a traffic jam on a motorway, it gets blocked and everything slows down. When this occurs, the energy begins to push backwards and downwards. This blockage and then return of energy has a negative effect upon the body.

So how can we reverse this situation? The logical answer is to make our throat as big as our trunk. Now you are wondering how can we make the throat area as wide as the trunk?

The answer is simple, by making sounds. There is no specific sound. You can make any sound you like. If it's painful say "Ooh!", if it's pleasurable, say "Ahh..." Make any sound that feels right to you. You can even cry to open the throat and release the waves of sadness or scream with anger to disperse anger from your Throat Chakra. The point is to express the emotion and allow it to release through the throat via sound.

Allow yourself to experiment with a wide variety of sounds. Your voice should always be expressed, your throat open, allowing passage of energy through. This allows the energy from the pelvic area to travel upwards freely.

Interestingly enough, when you fully release sound in the form of loud expression and big sounds, what happens is that the energy travels outwards from your Throat Chakra creating a vacuum in the throat. When this vacuum is created, it pulls the energy from the pelvis to the throat. So this actually has a pulling effect on the energy.

Sound is a very important part of the emotional release process. We are afraid to make noises because the children or neighbours may hear us, but what we do when we silence ourselves is that we prohibit the energy to move as it should and thus we suppress the Throat Chakra. It is very important when we are orgasmic that the energy travels upwards and passes through the head. In Tantric Journey, we believe that energy passing through the head is the most important part of orgasm because of what occurs in the pineal gland. In terms of emotional release and full body healing, any orgasm below the throat is for sexuality only and not much use to full release and healing. When orgasmic energy fuses in the pineal gland which is in the 6th Chakra, it sends messages to activate stem cells in the body which does all the repairing and healing of all bodily functions.

The following are some sounds you can practice by yourself to open up your Chakras. Each sound resonates with its corresponding Chakra.

These are called Bija Mantras

Bija Mantra	Chakra
Lam	Root
Vam	Sacral
Ram	Solar Plexus
Yam	Heart
Ham	Throat
Om or Ksham	Third Eye
Om or Silence	Crown

Smell

It is commonly recognised that bears have a highly developed sense of smell and can detect food from a great distance away, however, the importance of the human sense of smell has been underestimated. Humans and other primates have been regarded as primarily 'optical animals' with highly developed powers of vision but an undeveloped sense of smell. It is widely overlooked that humans use olfactory communication and are even able to produce and perceive certain pheromones and that pheromones play an important role in the behavioural and reproductive biology of humans.

Whilst looks might appear to be the most important factor at the start of any relationship, it is usually the 'look' of someone that is the initial cue to strike up a possible relationship, but what drives the strong emotional feelings are a series of chemical signals being emitted by the male. These chemical signals known as pheromones, interact with specific sites in female nostrils to cause intense emotional feelings.

This highly complex sense of smell is held by human females to ensure the production of genetically diverse offspring allowing her to select the best partner for producing strong children.

The pheromones originate in the apocrine glands (sweat glands) in humans. These glands are focused in areas around the face, chest, armpits, groin etc. and wherever body hair exists, and become activated after puberty when the search for a mate begins. The Greek word pheromone means to transfer and excite which demonstrates how key smell is in sensuality.

I stress to my clients that smell is important in the quest of finding a mate. Think about a time when you walked by a man and could smell a cologne that a loved one used to wear all the time. Chances are it evoked powerful and positive feelings of nostalgia. When the smell gateway is blocked by negative energy, it can become difficult for my clients to engage in a healthy relationship with a compatible mate.

To help release the negative energy that is blocking this gateway, I have my clients smell every part of the body gently, not sexually. This is conscious smelling, which means that I want my clients to be focused on it through the entire process. If I'm holding a couples session, each person will take turns as a giver and a receiver.

If a client feels difficulty while engaging in this breathing exercise, she needs to keep engaging in focused breathing and smelling for the negative energy to be released from her gateway. Only then is it possible to replace this negative energy with the positive energy that's necessary for establishing a loving and beneficial relationship. I've found that this is one of the most popular exercises for couples to engage in during sessions, as smell can be very arousing when negativity leaves the gateway.

Taste

Taste is a very powerful energy centre within our bodies, which means that this is a particularly powerful gateway.

There are five main tastes: sweet, sour, salty, bitter and astringent and each has its own set of sensors on different parts of the tongue that is connected to a different part of the brain. Stimulating these sensors is a wonderful way to energise our minds and our bodies.

During the Tantric Journey Bodywork, I have my client taste her partner's whole body in a way that isn't sensual, but conscious. For example, if you're focused on hearing what another person has to say to you, you're consciously listening to them. Tasting merely means that you're paying attention to how different parts of your partner's body taste, all while focusing on your breathing exercises.

If this is the gateway that's blocked up, the client will notice that she'll begin to feel emotional as she tastes different parts of the body. This is when the energy is being released from the gateway, allowing the client to discover a new type of sense that enables her to connect with her partner in new and intimate ways.

Holistic Body Therapy

Before continuing to explore the Tantric Journey healing process and the seven energy centres (or Chakras), it's important for clients to note that there's a key difference between a Lover and a Healer. Both are opening the same Chakra channel; however, the intention and direction will be different based on the person. A Healer will do so to release negative energies from the body, while the Lover will do this to infuse the physical self with positive energy.

Holistic Body Therapy, unlike a massage treatment, treats your whole body, mind and spirit based on ancient Tantric Philosophy. Treatment entails Deep Bodywork, stretching the body into yoga postures, lifting, rocking, and coaching on breathing, sound, body movement and pelvic floor exercises.

Treatment is based on the balancing of vibrational energies of the seven major Chakra points, which are located in the crown, forehead, throat, heart, solar plexus, sacrum and the perineum. Chakras act as a pump to move energies throughout the body, and the same must be energetically positive to be active.

Chakras can become energetically negative due to traumas, accidents, abuse, stresses of life, and religious and cultural beliefs. In this case the negative Chakras are unable to move the energies effectively; the results can often include dysfunctions, illness, and disease. The Holistic Body-Mind Therapy treatment is intended to heal the Chakras by creating and moving positively charged Life Force energies from the Sacrum to Crown.

When the positive energy meets up with the negative energy centres' in the body, it can transform a negative Chakra into a more positive state. During this process, lifelong emotional and physical blocks and wounds can be healed.

Understanding the Chakras: what is their purpose?

Before I explain what the Chakras are associated with, their purpose and how I clear the Chakras as part of my work, I wish to draw a distinction between primary and secondary Chakras, as these often become confused. I deal with the primary Chakras which are the inner Chakras, i.e. the Chakras described by the original Tantra. The West tends to be more familiar with secondary Chakras as this is the commonly used system in the New Age movement and the system usually shown in Western literature and taught in Western schools. Unlike the primary Chakras, the secondary Chakras are shown to have a specific form (usually described as vortexes of energy); they have a colour attributed to them and a specific precise location in the auric body. Primary Chakras are located in the etheric body.

The Seven Primary Chakras	
Chakra No.	**Associated with**
Chakra one	Survival, trust and safety
Chakra two	Emotions and sexuality
Chakra three	Power, will and intimacy

Chakra four	**Love and balance**
Chakra five	**Communication and creativity**
Chakra six	**Intuition, awareness and imagination**
Chakra seven	**Knowledge, understanding and spirituality**

"Chakra", which means "wheel" in Sanskrit, can be simply described as centres of energy that permeate the entire body along the length of the spine. Interestingly, the spacing of Chakras matches the location of major endocrine centres in the body. The Chakras can become easily blocked causing imbalance and disease.

Initiating Love and Intimacy Through the Chakras

You are designed to experience real and authentic love

The concept of Chakras is rooted in the mind/body connection — or, more accurately, the spirit/body connection and through understanding your Chakras you can begin to implement positive change in your life. When a person is unbalanced in their Chakras, you'll hear them using expressions such as, "I'm having an off day," or "Nothing seems to be going right today." (Chakra imbalance is similar to hormone imbalance as Chakras are located parallel to hormone-producing glands). Whereas if the Chakras are balanced, you'll hear expressions like, "I've had a great day," or "everything has just slotted into place today". This sense of harmony comes when everything is lined up and the energy is flowing throughout your whole body. This sense of harmony and positivity can be extended to all areas of your life including your love life.

You should strive to achieve a positive energy state for all your Chakras, which will then aid you in attracting a suitable partner with a magnetic-like energy field. To be receptive to finding a soul-mate, you need to open your Crown Chakra first and this will bring you into contact with a person with whom you can connect with on an emotional, spiritual and physical level.

Once you have found someone you feel you have a connection with, and then you need to open your Third-eye Chakra, and see the person fully for who they really are. If you like what you see, then you can open your Throat Chakra, and talk with that person. You need to spend a long time talking and communicating and all of this is before any physical relationship has formed. If you talk long enough then you will truly and authentically fall in love. It is a matter of dedicating time to each level and allowing the relationship to develop. As lovers you will open and communicate with the Chakras from the crown downwards and you will consolidate with each other on each level, synchronising with each other as you move through the Chakras.

If you like what you hear, then you can open your Heart Chakra. If love is felt, then you can open your Solar Plexus Chakra- meaning that you can touch the other person and be intimate exploring all five sensors as a giver and a receiver, but still without having sex. All the time, this is about taking time and communicating with each other on every single level.

If you like what you feel, and then finally you can open up your Sex Chakra and experience spiritual sex which is felt throughout the whole body and in every Chakra point, connecting two people on every level -- physically, emotionally and spiritually. By the stage of sexual intercourse, you'll already be connected on emotional and spiritual planes and will have fallen in love at a deeper level.

The final stage of this journey is to open the first Base Chakra and to live happily ever after.

Lover and Healer, both work on opening the same Chakra path, but with a different intention. Lover's intention is to meet the partner in a spiritual space and to form a lifelong relationship to provide safety and security. As a Healer my intention is to meet the client in a safe, sacred space and to help her to connect with spirituality. So the lover and the healer work on opposite directions of the same Chakra chart for different intentions.

As a healer I do not want clients to fall in love with me as they would with a partner. I do not wish to form deep loving relationships with them as a soul mate, so I do not treat their Chakras from the crown downwards as a lover would, but instead I work upwards from the base, restoring energetic balance on every level and releasing negative emotion by drawing sexual energy, (life's force), upwards from the Base Chakra throughout their system. I am working as a therapist and my aim is to release negative emotion and restore the body's natural state of bliss. Over a series of sessionswhich take place over a period of time, a mutually trusting working relationship is able to grow. As my clients shed their emotional trauma and work through their emotional blockages they will eventually no longer need to see me as they usually meet the partner of their dreams or transform their existing relationship.

Clearing the Chakras

When I am treating a client I work on each Chakra individually and help to move blockages from each energy centre. It is common for me to find the following emotions held in the Chakras:

1. Fear: this is often felt when the client feels her survival is threatened. She fears for her life; she fears she will not survive.
2. Guilt: this keeps us trapped. It stops us from connecting with others and prevents the full potential of emotional bonds with others being created.
3. Shame: is the enemy of spontaneity, creativity, self-esteem, and personal empowerment.
4. Grief: is a heavy burden to carry. It hinders the love and lightness that can be experienced.
5. Lies: Misinformation hinders our relationship to the world and distorts the thinking and the ultimate actions of the person who hears the lie and of the person who tells it.
6. Illusion: This is a form of crooked thinking. By hiding away from reality and not seeing the big picture, your perception of life will be hindered.
7. Attachment: Holding on to things that no longer serve their purpose and focusing all of one's attention in one area can mean that your perception becomes distorted and your ability to resolve matters is impaired. When you release the stagnant emotions, you will definitely feel less troubled and more inclined to let go and move on.

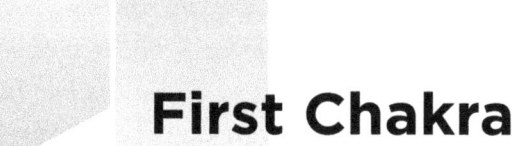

First Chakra

Each Chakra has a role to perform, same as each hormone producing gland. So let's start with the First Chakra, which is known as the Base Chakra, or the Root Chakra. This represents your confidence, your security, your safety, your trust, and other positive emotions. When my clients come to me, the first thing is that they notice that I am a man, and more often than not, they've been damaged by a man. I represent all men in their minds, so they are very suspicious about me.

What I have to do is then start opening the First Chakra by talking to her, by listening to her and answering her questions. Basically what I am doing in the first session and only in the first few hours when a new client comes to me is opening the First Chakra by communicating without even touching.

When I talk to them, I am earning their trust with what I have to say because if the client accepts what I say, they begin to trust me and then they will ask me more questions. If I am able to answer these questions to their satisfaction, then they are going to trust me even more. The first few hours a treatment is focused upon earning a client's trust and allowing her to relax and be comfortable in the space that I am working in and to develop a connection. Only when that is achieved can we move forward in the healing process so that Bodywork can begin. Every client is different because every client's block is unique. I have to accept her, whoever she is, and wherever she is in at that particular time, as this is essential to the healing process. The purpose of this Talking therapy is to open her mind in order to earn sufficient trust to get permission to access her body. I also offer this service via a Skype session from anywhere in the world which is very healing for a woman.

I work without pre-judgements, whenever a client comes to me, because I really don't know what I need to do unless I've interacted with the client's emotions. They are not constant. They keep changing over time. Their thoughts change; their feelings change; their emotions change; and everything changes like the waves of the sea. So I need to keep up with that to feel into their energy, like riding a wave, rather than change them. Nobody can change or fix a woman. They have to change themselves. So I am just like a facilitator to help the woman understand and accept the trauma that she has been through. There is no time limit for this work. You cannot rush as rushing will only facilitate blockages in the client; in this process it is true that time is a great healer. Everything has to be on the client's terms, not my terms or a set schedule. There are certain fundamental things that I follow as a therapist. When a client comes to me, I identify an intention. Intention and intent are the keys to all healing. If you can get the intent right, everything else will follow. Before I start a healing session, I make sure my healing intent is clear: it's clearly formed and it is focused. I am then guided by what I need to do, and everything else unfolds from this intent. This is the first stage of creating the healing process.

Once I have formed the intent, I focus very strongly on that intention. Once I focus on that intention then everything works automatically. I don't even have to try anything, but that is my intention and everything works into the right place.

"You are what your deepest desire is.
As your desire is, so is your intention.
As your intention is, so is your will.
As your will is, so is your deed.
As your deed is, so is your destiny."
- Principal Upanishads

Women are more sensitive than men because historically they had to protect themselves from external feelings; this means that they are sensitive and always on guard much more than men. They are more fearful. They are more shamed. They are guiltier when feeling pleasure. They get angrier quickly and they get sad quickly. So they are basically an emotional-minded body whereas the man is not. Man is a logical body. That does not mean women are not logical, or men are not emotional, please don't get me wrong. Women are logical in their masculine part of the body and men are emotional in their feminine part of the body.

Therefore I use my feminine energy to connect with women at the beginning and then use my masculine energy during the treatment to heal women. It is important for a healer to have this ability to change from masculine to feminine and vice versa when dealing with victims suffering from trauma especially as a result of men. Women need to feel that they are with another woman and not with a man. They need to feel the feminine touch initially in order to feel safe.

The idea here is to teach my clients that not all men are bad. Imagine when they were in their childhood, and they burned themselves on an iron and their first thought is that they should never touch another iron again. So they will never touch any iron, even when they grow up because it is in their cellular memory. But if somebody can show them that there are so many irons with warm and different temperatures, they can actually change the way they think and act on certain things. I give them the positivity and trust that they need to see that not all men are bad, so they can start breaking away from their past.

CASE STUDY

"I came across Mal about 15 years ago whilst researching what healers there were in the UK working with Brandon Bay's Journey Therapy methods. I knew I had a lot of issues, I was closed sexually and ashamed of myself. I dressed provocatively and used my sexuality to get the love I was seeking. I slept with so many men just for the game of it. All sexual encounters were a play that may have looked sexy on the outside, but on the inside I was numb and disconnected. I had cancerous cells forming in my cervix and I knew I needed healing. Although I had read up about Mal's Tantric Journey work, I really didn't know what to expect.

During the first session we did a meditation that involved sitting in silence with eye contact (eye gazing meditation). Instead of being able to receive his loving gaze I felt total distrust and when he touched me (with most of my clothes on at this stage) I couldn't receive it as all I felt was this distrust. I decided not to go back again and over the next year I began to work on myself, going to healing groups and seeing energy healers. I began to realize the distrust I had felt wasn't to do with Mal, it was my own distrust. I felt ready to face it and see Mal again, with the determination that this time I wouldn't run away no matter what.

I went on a long healing journey with Mal. The tightness, ticklishness, pain, the anger, rage, shame and emotional agony were all revealed and released as this incredible man touched me, held, caressed and healed me. Although I was beginning to understand some of the things that had resulted in this pain, in a way it didn't matter what the stories were, what mattered was that I was willing to feel it. And through deep yoni healing was able to release years of anger that had turned to numbness. I began to experience the connection between love and sex, my body opening and female ejaculation (a healing orgasmic release of amrita). Each time I released like this I would open to a deeper level of pain and endless tears until eventually, only love and pleasure and grace were left. Mal was always there holding, caressing, loving me every step of the way.

Learning to receive was one thing, but there was also learning how to give. Once I could connect to the pleasure in my body, I could give from that place, and enjoy touching a body including the yoni or lingam (penis) without feeling disgust or shame. It was such a new freedom in my life. I realized touching someone from a place of love and sexual connection within had the power to heal them.

I wanted to share what I had received from Mal with others and began to offer Tantric Healing sessions. Looking back, I think I went into it too soon and wasn't strong or grounded enough to be working as a sexual healer. But I learnt so much over the years and have since helped hundreds of people who wanted to free themselves of the pain that prevents them from being both loving and powerful in their sexuality.

After some years of not seeing Mal, I decided to see him again. I had changed a lot, the cancerous cells had gone and I was a much more genuine person, yet there was a deep longing to settle down and meet someone and it wasn't happening. The painful struggle to meet someone was actually preventing it from happening. I had closed down again. After a few sessions with Mal, I felt complete, joyful and opening. (I remember one of those sessions involved Mal resting his hand over my yoni while I fell into a dream like space, sometimes it's the simplest things!).

Shortly after these sessions I entered into a serious relationship with a long term friend who for many years I had resisted (as he hadn't fit the picture in my head of the man I would be with). He's now my husband and the love of my life.

I was physically shut down when I first met Mal and through his healing I changed profoundly. Yet the journey continues; I'm still growing, I still close occasionally, I'm still learning, but these days it's so much easier to open up again and return to what feels good. Mal showed me what it feels like to be in bliss, peace, to feel safe, to be loved and honoured like every woman should be; her yoni, toes, breasts, fingertips - her entire body. He loved me enough until I was able to do it myself."

- R. N. December, 2013

Second Chakra

The Second Chakra is the Sex Chakra which surprisingly isn't more difficult to open than the First Chakra. Getting someone to trust you takes a considerable amount of time and effort, especially if a client has been hurt by a man before. I could open a Sex Chakra within the first day for a client, but it might take me weeks to open up that First Chakra and get her to trust me. Once I've opened up the First Chakra, only then can I proceed on and open up the Sex Chakra.

To open up the Sex Chakra, I can't tell my client to take her clothes off and let me do a Yoni massage. It doesn't happen like that. So first of all I explain to her the features and benefits of the treatment, then she goes through a cleansing ritual by having a steam - shower. This cleaning process is important because washing your body cleanses all the negative energy that you have on your aura and your body. Then she comes to me to be taught some yogic body movements, meditations, pelvic floor exercises, breathing techniques and how to make sounds (mantras). This can help her understand the importance of breathing deeply, making sounds and moving the body, when I am giving her a massage.

During these rituals, the client will begin to slowly open up to me even before I begin touching her. We do some pelvic squeezes to open the PC muscles (pubococcygeus muscle) around the Yoni area. Throughout the entire time, I will explain to the client how and why these things need to be done, just so she can feel more confident and trusting of me.

After that, I massage the client with whatever level of comfort she wants; in other words, she can keep her clothes on, she can wear her underwear, or she can completely remove her clothing. During this time, I also tell her that her clothes represent certain emotions. For example, if I massage a client fully clothed, then each layer may represent some shame, fear, sadness, guilt, mistrust, anger and so forth.

For example her bra could be representative of some form of guilt or self-consciousness while the underwear could represent fear or shame. These clothes represent different emotions, so I slowly help her build up the confidence she needs to peel these layers back until she's comfortable with herself. This is like peeling an onion layer; however, I'm always respectful if a client wants to remain clothed during a massage. The goal isn't to rush the healing process; it's to do it at a pace that's comfortable for the client.

On the first day of opening up the Sex Chakra, I will only massage her with her clothes on, because this gives me an idea of what emotions and traumas she's been burdened with. If I try to move the process too fast, she might become scared and not want to engage in the healing process altogether. This creates a trustful relationship, because I demonstrate that I'm able to respect her boundaries, and she learns how to vocalize her comfort levels. The next time she comes to me, I'll tell her to keep on whatever clothes she wants, but to be mindful that they represent an emotion. If she wants to peel away that emotion, she can do so by removing a specific clothing item from her body. During the next session, she might be able to remove her bra; during the next, she might feel comfortable taking off her pants. I'm always vocal about what areas I'm going to massage so that she never feels as though her body isn't being respected. When she's able to expose her whole body to me, I've earned all of her trust, as she no longer feels the shameful or guilty emotions that were represented by her clothing.

Once the layers of emotions are helped to remove at the clothing level, my next task is to help the client to move on to peel off deeper layers of emotions from the body at three levels: skin level, extrinsic muscular level and intrinsic muscular level.

Once she takes off all of her clothes, I do a full body massage. I don't touch the genital area, as I want her to experience a full body massage without any clothes on for her to be able to relax into a massage. If I touch the genital area too soon, she'll lose all trust in me. The longer it takes to get to that point, the better, because it means she's built up a significant level of trust in me.

The whole goal is to get the client to open up in a way that makes her feel comfortable, not vulnerable. Some clients ask me to remove their clothing for them during the massage, but I can't do that because that's not conducive to the healing process. The client is the one who has to peel back the onion, not me. Only then can she relax into a full body massage without feeling shameful or fearful of a man.

Once I'm engaging in the body massage, the client will start to awaken and engage with the movements; in other words, she's becoming aroused. The whole massage itself takes about three hours to complete, because it's one-third slower than the typical massage you receive at a beauty salon or a spa. The reason for this slowness and depth is that it evokes the negative emotions that have been buried in the cellular memory.

At the end of my three-hour massage, the client is usually in a deep trance. This is when I keep one hand above the yoni and one hand above the crown, and I wake her up to ask her if I can do a yoni massage. If she says yes, I tell her that if at any stage she feels uncomfortable she is to let me know and I will stop the yoni massage. So I carry on with the yoni massage with continuous permission sought from time to time as she could withdraw the permission due to the evoking of past traumas.

While I'm doing the yoni massage, I tell the client how I'm going to touch her, why I'm touching her this way, and why I see the yoni as the same as any other part of the body. This can help my client feel more comfortable during the yoni massage. I've done over 3,000 yoni massages, so my clients know that I don't see this as a sexual act; in fact, it's a lot like going to the gynaecologist.

When I'm massaging the yoni, I'm ensuring that I massage all the pressure points, which are the knots that are blocking the energy flow into the yoni. This is like a deep tissue massage that you would experience on your neck or on the back of the head. When I massage the yoni, it can be painful sometimes, but then I massage the C-spot (Clitoris) of the yoni to dilute the physical and / or emotional pain to help her let go of her nervousness and distrust. Sometimes a lot of shame shuts down the yoni, then I massage the yoni lips gently where most of the shame is stored and the shame dissipates. Meanwhile, I encourage the client to continue to focus on her breathing so she can release her negative energy; after all, if she's holding onto her breath, she can't release her emotions. I know when my clients aren't breathing, because we're connecting as one person during the massage. I'll feel her breath get shallow, which means she's stopped focusing on letting out her negative energies. If a client stops breathing deeply, I'll start breathing for her to remind her to stay focused on her breath. At this point, I ask the client if she's ready and open, and if she gives me permission, I'll start massaging the inner part of the yoni. I always talk to my clients through this process, because the yoni massage is very unique, and not everyone experiences it.

As you can see in the diagram below yoni holds emotions in different places and when you massage these points gently incorporating breath, the negative emotions just transform into positive emotions and pleasure within a very short time. The whole process is to remove negative imprints externally first and then to move on to yoni internally. It is these stagnant emotions in the yoni that block your sexuality, orgasmic potential, relationships, health and happiness.

Yoni Emotions Storage Locations

Pubic Bone

G Spot
Faking orgasm, performance, anxiety, feeling inadequate

Clitoris
Nervousness, Distrust, impatience, holding tight

Vaginal Lips
Fear of opening, shame, desire to hide

Vaginal Canal
Anger, neediness, abortions & childbirth traumas

Perineum and Perineal Sponge
Difficulty letting go, numbness

The Yoni has got four different points or buttons. The day you were born, all these buttons were positive, pure, innocent, and loving and pleasurable. But after you were born, during whatever experience you had as a child, trauma or what you have seen, what happened to you, what you heard, what you have read and what you saw on the TV, all these things collectively produce emotions such as fear, shame, guilt etc., which get stored in the yoni at cellular level and transform these positive cells into emotional negative cells.

Yoni Healing Through 4 Types Of Body Cells

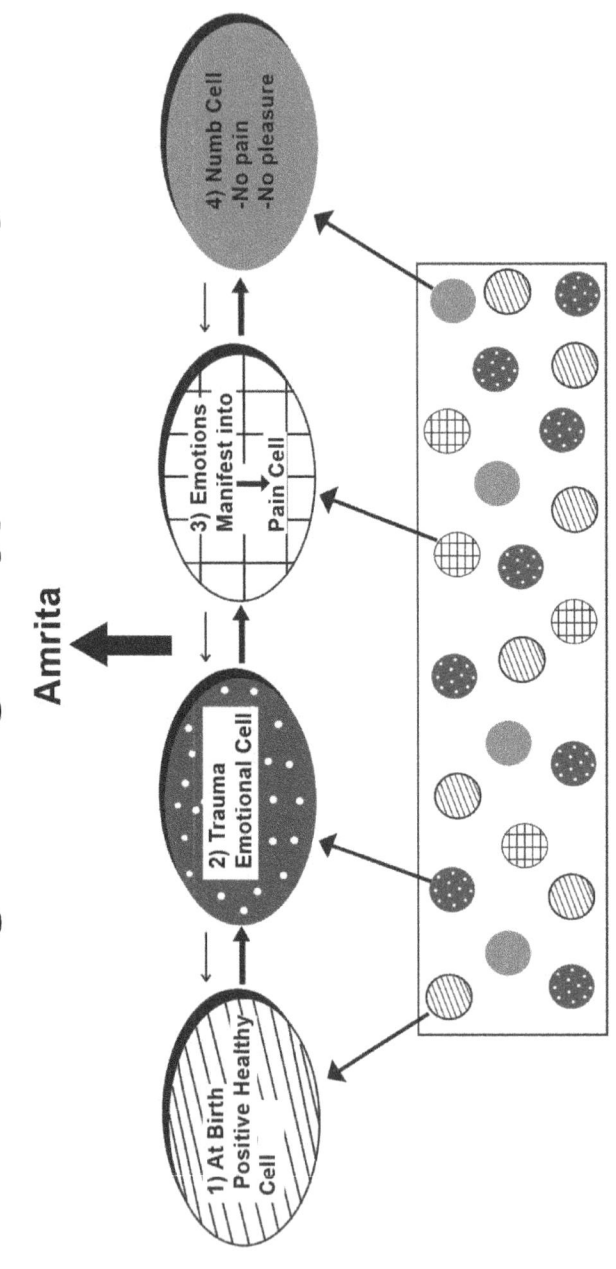

Yoni = Female Prostate

1) At Birth Positive Healthy Cell

2) Trauma Emotional Cell

3) Emotions Manifest into Pain Cell

4) Numb Cell
-No pain
-No pleasure

Amrita

Now this pleasure button in the yoni can then become an emotional button as a result of trauma. Now you have this second type of button in the yoni – emotional buttons. As you grow up, emotional buttons are left ignored, which means they often manifest into physical pain buttons. Therefore the yoni starts to feel pain, especially if you're beginning to have sex.

All these stored emotions are in the yoni cellular memory and, as emotions manifest into physical pain, you will feel this physical pain. Physical pain is there to communicate to you that you need to do something about healing your yoni. It's a lot like how the body reminds us if we're not getting enough sleep or if we're constantly stressed out by giving us headaches. So it's the body's way of communicating with you to change whatever you are doing to make you happy. Otherwise, you become unhappy.

Sometimes women have sex without foreplay or preparation, which can be traumatising to the woman in the area of the yoni. I should probably explain here that the woman and the yoni in Tantric are defined as two different entities. The voice is given to yoni and if the yoni feels as though you're not doing anything to make this pain go away, to relieve the pain it is suffering, it's going to enter the fourth stage, which involves feeling numbness or sexually "shutting down" on you.

When I'm massaging the yoni, my clients react differently based on the combination of buttons they have in the yoni. Some clients won't feel anything because their buttons are numb; others will feel emotional because they have emotional buttons. So my task is really to convert those numb buttons into pleasure buttons. To do that, it has to go through the pain and the emotions before it can receive pleasure. It's the same pathway from pleasure to emotion, emotion to pain, and pain to numbness so the reversal has to go to exactly the same pathway, but in the opposite direction. It is not possible to bypass the pain and the emotion to achieve pleasure.

Yoni massage is done in a very slow motion, like a snail on the yoni; if there is too much friction, the yoni can shut down. So when massaging so slowly and gently, with a feminine touch, the yoni starts opening up and a time comes that the yoni opens further so you can massage deeper and harder, using a masculine touch. As a healer I have learned to oscillate between the masculine and feminine energies within me. My left hand is the feminine hand and the right hand is the masculine. I start with my feminine left hand and change into my masculine right hand at the end of the yoni massage

To help describe the numbness, imagine that there's an egg inside the yoni and the eggshell is very thin the day you were born. If you have cracked this eggshell it will break and the water will fully come out which we call in Sanskrit "amrita," or female ejaculation. But what happens in the yoni is that this eggshell gets thicker and thicker and thicker because of trauma and emotions. So as you grow up, this eggshell is not something that you can tap to release Amrita, because it's like a steel eggshell. Each trauma in the yoni makes this egg shell go harder and harder. It also gets harder as you get older.

So by doing a gentle and slow massage, you can transform the eggshell from a very thick steel to a normal eggshell. During the yoni massage, a time will come when just a slight press on the yoni's eggshell will cause it to burst, or ejaculate from the sacred space of the woman. When this liquid comes out you will start releasing emotions. I term this stage as "Yoni Crying". During this stage clients may also shiver and tremble for up to an hour, this is called Kundalini Awakening. Body shaking is a way of dispersing stagnant negative emotions (the same process that Dr Peter Levine refers to in his study) from the body, making way for orgasmic positive energy to flow freely from the pelvic to the crown to feel a full body orgasm in the head. The body also flexes at this stage backwards and forward arching in and out, making very loud sounds and screaming and breathing deeply. When this process is taking place I observe and hold the space to the woman to open up freely like a beautiful lotus flower.

As you release emotions, after a few minutes, you will feel so much pleasure in your body, not just in the yoni, but like an electric current going through the body. This is really not even like an orgasm, according to my clients. What a few clients have said, is that before treatment they felt like they had a lot of lead inside their body and that after the treatment this lead had gone (in the form of liquid) and they suddenly felt very light, peaceful, and loving. At this point, my clients have met the goddesses within them, and you can tell: they look, ten to twenty years younger in their face.

It's a real privilege to see this happen, because for a moment, you see a client manifest and become the goddess within herself. It is truly amazing to witness this goddess-like face in this moment of ecstasy.

So once this happens, the Second Chakra has opened, which means you can go deeper to release even more emotions. If it's their first time ejaculating, though, I usually stop there, because I don't want to overwhelm them with emotions. I usually make a judgment call at the time, based on how my client is feeling throughout the healing process. So this is the process of the opening the Second Chakra.

Opening the Sex Chakra is nothing or very little to do with sex. It is an emotional release treatment. When you start awakening and arousing a woman you have to first release the very emotions that are blocking her arousal and the orgasm. If a woman can't have an orgasm, she's usually sad or angry. That's why we need to focus on her anger and sadness, because it helps her connect with her Chakra so she can release it. Once she does that, the orgasm usually happens by itself. That's why this isn't a sexual treatment; it's an emotional release treatment.

As soon as you say it's a sexual healing treatment, you'll find that many women will be afraid to engage in it because the word "sex" is what caused them the original trauma. This is especially true when they see that a man will be providing the yoni massage, because a man equals sex, and sex equals pain. So it's important for people to realize that this isn't about sex; it's about releasing a negative emotion that's stored within your body. Once you get rid of that emotion, most of my clients have very good orgasms with their partner that they never before had. It's an empowering treatment that lasts a lifetime.

CASE STUDY

When Tina came to me she was complaining of severe miserable perimenopausal symptoms. She explained to me how she had lack of energy, no motivation and a lack of libido. At only 49 years of age she had so many aches and pains that she described herself as 'being spent'; she was riddled with guilt about overspending and said that on the rare occasions she did have sex she found it impossible to orgasm. She described how she felt that she was "spiralling downwards" and had no energy left to fight. For Tina life was just one big chore. With horrific cramps and her weight gain despite her best efforts to maintain her figure she felt depressed and as if she had achieved nothing in life.

When I started treating Tina I found that she had blockages in her Sacral Chakra; this is the seat of emotions. It is the home of passion, imagination, motivation and creativity; her blockages were causing her to feel dull and depressed. She was disconnected and blocked in this area because she was supressing her emotions due to past trauma and this was affecting her present relationships.

Over a series of one-to-one sessions I treated Tina and, through Tantric Journey therapy, her blockages were released allowing her to be free from pain and lethargy. She described how she felt 'alive' for the first time in years and with the Sacral Chakra functioning once more, she suddenly felt energised and her relationships improved dramatically. She not only went on to experience orgasms with her husband but was able to experience multi orgasmic response.

SIGNS OF A BALANCED SECOND CHAKRA

Easy Going
Expressive
Passionate
Creative
Emotionally Secure

Sense of love
Sexually Fulfilled
Filled with Joy
Warmth

SYMPTOMS OF AN IMBALANCED SECOND CHAKRA

Obsessions
Addictions
Creative blocks
Impotence
Promiscuity
PMT
Guilt
Depression
Hormonal imbalances
Lower back pain
Kidney stones
Urinary problems

Gynaecological issues
Lethargy
Prostate problems
Poor sense of taste
Self-hate
Manipulative
Oversensitive
Sexual dysfunction
Anger
Depression
Despair

Third Chakra

Once I've opened up the Sex Chakra, I work on the Third Chakra. Not surprisingly, a lot of people have blockages in the Third Chakra area, because it represents our intimacy. It is one of the most difficult Chakras to work with, as it's surrounded with many different emotions. When this chakra is blocked, this essentially means that the client is having trouble being truly intimate with another person. This doesn't mean in the sexual sense; this means being with someone and connecting with them heart, mind, body and soul.

The Third Chakra, intimacy Chakra, has five gateways which are represented by the five senses. One is touch, which means that the client is scared of being touched and / or to touch others intimately. The second is smell, which means that the client is scared of being smelled or unable to recognise the smell of her ideal partner due to desensitising the sense of smell. The third is hearing because the client is afraid of communicating. The fourth is taste, because the client is afraid of tasting someone and / or being receptive to someone tasting her. The fifth and final one is sight, because the client is afraid to see things as they are, within an intimate relationship. Fear or seeing eye-to-eye.

You don't always have to be scared of giving to have trouble with intimacy; many of my clients freely give, only to have trouble receiving intimacy. If there are five gateways, this means that there are ten different entrances for these five senses. All of these entrances have the potential to be blocked, which is why this Chakra can be one of the hardest to open. To determine which one it is, I'll typically use the exercises that I listed in the section on gateways. Over a period of time, I'll discover what's blocked so that we can remove the negative energy, thus replacing it with positive energy and intimacy.

CASE STUDY

When Jenny came to see me she had been recommended by a friend and admitted that she came out of desperation, because she 'couldn't bear to live her life the way it was any longer'. Jenny had been repeatedly complaining to her Doctor of low self-esteem, insecurity and of intimacy issues. She had been prescribed a series of different anti-depressants and had seen a string of counsellors and, although she had been desperate for them to work, nothing had ever worked on a long term basis.

She was on her third marriage and the fear of that coming to an end was the catalyst for her to come and see me. When I started to treat Jenny, the reason for her fear of intimacy and the issues she had experienced in all of her marriages became apparent for she had a blocked Solar Plexus Chakra. It took time to clear her blockages but, after coming to me for a number of sessions, she reported how she had gained trust in her marriage and had stopped suffering from jealousy and insecurity. Her marriage started to get back on track and she explained how she was no longer worried about hanging on to her husband because she suddenly felt self-sufficient in a confident and positive way.

SIGNS OF A BALANCED THIRD CHAKRA

Feeling secure
Flexibility
Well Nourished
Healthy Weight
Feeling at ease
Strong Will Power
Discernment

SYMPTOMS OF AN IMBALANCED THIRD CHAKRA

Control issues
Stomach ulcers
Diabetes
Pancreatitis
Indigestion
Eating disorders
Colon diseases
Anger/irritability
Lack of self-esteem
Insecurity
Lethargy

Fourth Chakra

After the Intimacy Chakra is the Heart Chakra. People are very scared to open the heart for a multitude of reasons, perhaps their father left the house when they were a child. The masculine energy that she loved is lost, so she wants to protect her heart by not opening the heart in case this damage happens again. Or perhaps the father abused her when she was a child, and this shut her heart and lost trust and love in the most trusted masculine person in her life. Maybe her first boyfriend let her down, broke her heart, or the first husband broke her heart.

Shutting a woman's heart is a way of protecting herself, so that she will not be subject to the same damage again. That's why the opening of the Heart Chakra is more difficult than opening the Intimacy Chakra or the Sex Chakra or the First Chakra. That's why I have to teach my clients some essential lessons. There are two types of love people have. In most relationships people love because they say "if you love me, I will love you." This is known as conditional love, which means that when you don't get what you expected, you'll get hurt and shut your heart.

I teach my clients how to love unconditionally and without any expectations. I do this by loving my client unconditionally without expecting anything in return.

I'm not expecting her for emotional support. I'm not expecting sex from her. I'm not expecting money from her. I'm not expecting anything from her. Instead I'm treating her with my total love, unconditional love. When she feels that unconditional love, then she will learn to give that unconditional love to me – and once she learns how to love one man, she can go on to love another in a beautiful and trusting relationship as she will know that no unconditional love can hurt her and with this knowledge she will be able to open her heart fully.

When a woman knows how to unconditionally love someone, she can't ever get hurt because she won't be expecting something from that other person. Once she understands this, she'll be more interested in unconditional love because she'll find it to be safer. The ultimate goal is to have her opening up her heart for love, so the energy will start flowing through the heart.

You need to have a heart to be in any relationship or to enjoy your job or have friendships; without the heart, you can't do anything but be a robot.

CASE STUDY

"I believe we are finally on the right track. When my husband massaged me, his intention was to release any blocks. He did a lot of internal massage which was uncomfortable, even painful in places and he could feel a lot of the ridges in my yoni softening. I focused on working with my breath, which helped me through the discomfort. Afterwards, when we were making love, I had a huge emotional release which was centred in my Heart Chakra. It came with a burst of healing tears, and then I ejaculated twice. So, I think we did something correctly.

What is strange is that during our marriage, I have had some extraordinary sexually transcendent experiences. I have experienced a type or orgasm that you call the 'God orgasm' - where it did just happen, as you describe, and it came deep from my cervix and felt like every cell of my body was merging with the Universe. My frustration is that it happens so rarely. It is almost worse knowing that I am capable of it and yet not being able to reach it. My dream is to have access to that all of the time.

I have done a lot of yoga, meditation, and studied Tantra in the past. I am very familiar with the concept that the body stores all emotional traumas in our cells. Because I have a history of childhood sexual abuse, I have spent many years working to unlock and release that trauma.

It is strange to me that I suddenly had this sense of urgency that I had to connect more deeply with my full sexual potential. I am happy to keep exploring with my husband as it seems to be helping. Lovemaking felt much better after the ejaculation, but I still was not able to have an orgasm during intercourse. Your guidance has helped immensely and I know we are getting closer each day."

- C.O. February, 2013

Fifth Chakra

Perhaps the most difficult chakra to open is the Throat Chakra. There are no set rituals I use; I just get the client to talk through the yoni. I give a voice to the yoni that she never had before. This is very empowering for the woman. This is most common during the yoni massage, because this ritual encourages them to open up and start making noise. The yoni passes its energy up through the throat, and suddenly silent clients are screaming out very loudly and excitedly. This is because the throat chakra is open, which allows the client to have a full body orgasm.

When women have faced traumas in their lives – especially those of a sexual nature – it can be hard for them to open up this Chakra and let go. Perhaps it's because they've been told to be quiet and suffer in silence for so long that they feel this way. Also during trauma you experience an altered state of consciousness in a form of a frozen state (trance-like state). This freezes the vocals with negative emotions such as fear, shame, guilt etc. for the rest of your life, due to stuck energy in the Throat Chakra as they could not voice or react in response to the trauma. But when they go on the Tantric Journey, they're encouraged to connect their voice with mind, hearts, and body so that they're completely releasing the negative energy. When my clients have opened up their Throat Chakras, you can practically feel this negative emotion rushing out in terms of verbal anger, sadness etc. which means that my clients are ready to start the healing process.

Some signs that the Throat Chakra is out of balance are:

Difficulty expressing oneself
Poor learning ability
Lack of concentration
Habitual lying
Fear, doubt, uncertainty
Frightened to let go and make noise
Inability to experience a full body orgasm

CASE STUDY

The Fifth Chakra is one of the most fascinating and also one most likely to be blocked. Whilst referred to as the Throat Chakra it includes the neck, upper shoulders, the mouth, the jaw and the ears. This Chakra is the source of expression and a person who has a fully functioning Fifth Chakra will be able to speak their mind without forgetting their heart. They will be able to speak their truth without forgetting the feelings of others. People who are blocked here will live a lie, while a person with an open Chakra will live in their truth.

To date I have not met a client who is not carrying some tension in the neck, shoulders or jaw. Many of my clients have grown up with strict rules about how they should speak and behave in public: from a young age their freedom of speech has been supressed. On top of this, many children are raised 'to fit in' and 'not offend'. We are conditioned to hold back our words, lest we may offend someone. Under the burden of being unable to speak our mind, many people have lost their spontaneity, their zest for life and their voice.

I have treated thousands of women and most frequently I see blockages in the Fifth Chakra with symptoms ranging from shoulder pain, thyroid issues, problems speaking their mind or acute nose and throat problems. Once the Fifth Chakra is cleared, I find that clients can 'find themselves'; they are able to finally find their voice and their love of life returns. They can be comfortable with their own being and express themselves without fear or embarrassment.

RH 2013

Sixth Chakra

The next Chakra is your Third Eye Chakra, which is contained in the back of the head and in the pineal gland. This is where the positive energy within the body moves, flows, and fuses into the third eye. This is what helps my clients achieve full-body orgasms, because the positive energy finally completely enveloped their bodies. When you have your orgasm in the head, it fuses in the pineal gland. And then from there, in the pineal gland, it has the ability to send messages to every cell in our body to activate stem cells in every part of our body to activate our self-healing mechanism. Also this positive orgasmic energy has the ability to transform any negatively charged cells into positively charged cells. So any illnesses, any dysfunctions, any stress we have, any negative emotions, can get cleared with this orgasmic energy flow. Once it crosses through the third eye and into the crown of the head, this means that my client will be more enlightened and be a deeply spiritual person.

The primary function of the of female ejaculation is to get rid of the negative energies stuck in the body due to past trauma that block the positive orgasmic energy flow. The primary function of the female orgasm is to facilitate the body's self-healing repairing mechanism by activating our stem cells and immune system.

Women have so much power within them, and I feel privileged to be a part of that commitment to helping their minds, bodies and spirits awaken. Women are the people who need to awaken if they want to heal the world. Man's job is to stay in stillness and to create a sacred platform for the woman to open up like a beautiful flower. When this happens, the family unit gets better - your career, your relationship, your love life - everything gets better. Unfortunately this is not happening in the world and that's why we have wars. We have so many problems in every part of the world, so many illnesses. So many people are unhappy and suffering from emotional and physical traumas. The world is suffering as a result of this loss of role fulfilment. Unfortunately women have been put to sleep this way by the man and also it's a man who can awaken them

Five Signs your Sixth Chakra has Blockages:

1. You have an overriding sense of loss of direction. You don't feel you are on the right path. This sense of being lost and without inner guidance can lead to institutionalism, obsessively following a belief or putting rigid rules in place as a means of giving you a sense of purpose or meaning.

2. A negative imagination. Your mind is often focused on worries and regrets that are not founded. Regrets about the past and worries about the future often take centre stage. You imagine all the things that could go wrong, focus on all the negative things that could happen. You imagine that people think the worst of you and are often 'forced' into panic mode by the thought of the future.

3. You spend much of your day in analysing and over analysing mode. It is a strain trying to work everything out and make sense of everything and it causes you to get frustrated when you can't. You find it hard to turn off the analytical mode which results in a difficulty being present in the moment and can result in sleep pattern problems.

4. Life is a continual emotional roller coaster. You have a strong attachment to how you believe things should turn out and then suffer bitter disappointment when they don't go to plan.

You are fixed in how you believe things should be and become overly attached to plans.

5. You are prone to many of the following frequent/chronic complaints: headaches, upper/frontal sinus conditions, and neurological disorders, disorders of the eyes or ears, insomnia, lethargy.

Seventh Chakra

Opening the Crown Chakra is a lifelong process because it's a continuous opening. Because if I say that it takes only four petals to open the First Chakra, to open the Crown Chakra, you will need a thousand petals. So you can imagine how difficult that is to open the Crown Chakra. What's more, it's a lifelong pursuit that doesn't end once a client is done with my sessions. The more you open the Crown Chakra, the more spiritual the client becomes, the more empowered she becomes.

I'd like to explain what spiritual means to me because a lot of people think spirituality is a religion. Spirituality, for me, is not a religion, but it's a philosophy. I believe we are all made with positive and negative emotions. I believe if a person has less negative energy and more positive energy then that means less sadness, less fear, less anger, less greed is in the world, and it's been replaced with more happiness, more giving, and more love. I also believe that more pleasure in the body means that this person will be a positive being. For me, that means that a positive person will be more spiritual than a negative person. A non-spiritual person is angry, sad, greedy, or has a lot of negative energies in their body. Therefore, when I say that your Crown Chakra will take a long time to open, what I mean is as a woman, you must keep ejaculating regularly to get rid of your negative energies, all the way down from the Throat Chakra to the pelvic basin, cleansing you and detoxifying your negative emotions; in return, you create a vacuum that gets filled with positive energies.

So you become a more positive, loving, and peaceful person who is empowered in her own life.

Negative emotions create negative thoughts, negative feelings, negative actions and lose all sensations in the body to make it go numb and lose pleasure. Positive emotions create positive thoughts, positive feelings, positive actions and activate all bodily sensations to make the whole body pleasurable, ecstatic and bliss which is every woman's birth right.

As a result of that, this Crown Chakra will open and you will become an enlightened person. And it's as simple as that. It has nothing to do with being a religious person; it means being a spiritual, positive, and empowered human being.

Some signs that the Crown Chakra is out of balance are:

Co-ordination difficulties
Poor balance
Depression
Inability to learn
Sensitivity to light, sound, and environment
Fear of alienation/exclusion
Emotional rigidity
Clumsiness
Aversion to change
Lack of spiritual exploration

Breath Orgasm

For people who feel that they are already having a healthy orgasm, the following is a calculation to show the average person's orgasmic potential per one year:

Calculation To Show The Average Person's Orgasmic Potential Per One Year

Each healthy person's average orgasm lasts five waves = for 5 seconds

If a person makes love an average 2.3 times per week, during the 52 weeks in the year her orgasmic potential is as follows...

5 seconds X 2.3 per week X 52 weeks pa= 600 seconds (=under 10 minutes pa)

Tantra can transform this ability by many folds to help achieve an orgasm that can last for over 10 mins during any one session.

Tantric Journey can transform this ability by many folds to help achieve an orgasm that can last for over 10 minutes during any one session. It really is that powerful and incredible!

Breath orgasm works by removing negative emotions through breath and clearing the blocked energy pathway from the base of the spine to crown. It is this clearance that makes the orgasmic positive energy flow freely towards the crown and out of the body. It is a mind blowing experience!

Energy Orgasm

An orgasm is a positively-charged energy that needs to move throughout the body in order to produce the positive changes that are critical for Tantric Journey healing. For clients to understand the power of this energy, I always tell them not to think of an orgasm as a sexual thing, but as a form of energy. This means that an orgasm doesn't always have to be experienced from the yoni; it can be experienced in the head. Without even touching your yoni, you can experience a full-body orgasm.

Tasting, touching (physically or energetically), smelling, seeing, talking and hearing – all of these sensors can be opened to contribute to a lasting and exciting full-body energy orgasm. Energy orgasm doesn't require penetration; it just requires activating one of the senses that we've discussed throughout the course of this book.

Women are very lucky because they can have an orgasm in any part of the body. If a female client is connected to every part of her body, she'll be able to experience an orgasm in all these parts. If a woman can't, this means that she's feeling disconnected from her body. In other words, the fuse has blown; but when the wiring's connected again, then she can experience a full-body energy orgasm. This carries both good news and bad news with it. The good news is that women can have an orgasm anywhere in the body; the bad news, however, is

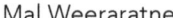

that it's much easier for women to get blocked by emotions because they're so sensitive and connected emotionally to all parts of the body. This means that women need to be wholly committed to connecting with their bodies, their Chakras, and their senses.

Body Orgasm and its Function

Orgasm Transforms Negative Cells into Positive Cells

Cell Receptors with molecules of Emotions

Positive Minds see an opportunity in every disaster

Negative Minds see a disaster in every opportunity

(+ve) Charged ORGASM

Rage

Fear

Greed

Cell

Anger

Mistrust

Guilt

Shame

Sad

Love

Positive Cell

Love

Happiness

Hypothalamus

Right thalamus

Kindness

Pleasure

Left thalamus

Compassion

Cerebellum

Now let's have a look at the function of the full body orgasm. Apart from pleasure and procreation, there are two main reasons for the full body orgasm. One is the healing and repairing potential, which I discussed above, by washing away the negative emotions through the positive orgasmic energy flow. The second most important reason is the hormonal chemical, where oxytocin that is released during the orgasm to bond with the partner who is facilitating this action. The Oxytocin Factor (Kerstin Uvnas-Moberg, 2003, Aspire, Scott Phelps, 2008), explains the purpose of oxytocin in detail. Here are just a few extracts from the text to further your understanding of the hormone dubbed the 'cuddle chemical' by some researchers:

"Oxytocin is a hormone that is released in a woman during childbirth, nursing a child, and during sexual activity. Commonly referred to as 'glue,' oxytocin creates a strong bond between the woman and the other involved. In the case of childbirth and nursing this bond is important because it creates a nurturing environment for the child. In a marriage relationship where sex is safe and beneficial, oxytocin helps keep the bond between a husband and wife strong. Outside of marriage however, the oxytocin bond can increase the emotional pain when the relationship has ended. Oxytocin is impartial. Whether during sexual activity between husband and wife or in a teenage romance, the hormone is still released and the bond is still created. Oxytocin promises an involuntary chemical commitment."

"Sex was created to unite two people, bringing a bond unlike any other relationship. This powerful bond is what sustains husband and wife until "death do us part" contributing to trust and security. Outside of marriage the release of oxytocin can lead to distrust, hostility, and insecurity. Sexual relationships without commitment still have a lasting bond. Oxytocin even has the power to sustain attachment within abusive relationships."

"Oxytocin also helps females bond with men. When a woman and man touch each other in a loving way, oxytocin is released in her brain. It makes her want more of that loving touch, and she begins to feel a bond with her partner. Sexual intercourse leads to the release of even more oxytocin, a desire to repeat the contact, and even stronger bonding.

"It is an involuntary process that cannot distinguish between a one-night stand and a lifelong soul mate. Oxytocin can cause a woman to bond to a man even during what was expected to be a short-term sexual relationship."

This explains what is missing in our society; women are bonding with men who have no intention of sticking around or raising any children that might result from the connection. While this may have had a biological necessity back in the caveman days, it's also causing women to become dependent on men who have no interest in being fulfilling and supportive partners. After making love a woman might mistake the oxytocin release for feelings that tell her, 'This is your Life partner.' Oxytocin is a hormone designed to bond partners through sex, so that they will create a family unit. The key to keep a man is to get him to release oxytocin every 3 days to keep up with the bonding. It's only a highly awake woman who could do this and not a woman who is sleeping and shut down due to her emotions and traumas. I must also add that female oxytocin bonding lasts for 21 days while man's bonding lasts only for 3 days.

What are the Benefits of Full Body Orgasm?

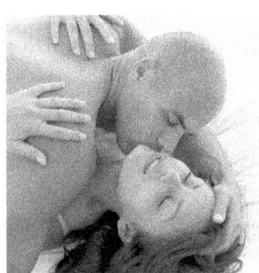

- Improves circulation to sexual organs helps with arousal disorders
- Helps to come out of Substance Dependency and saves Money
- Increases Life Span and helps Stay Young
- Emotional Detox process to Prevent Illnesses (Cancer) by transforming Negatively Charged Cells into Positively Charged Cells, creating an Alkaline Environment in the body
- Increases levels of Oxytocin Hormones to bond with the Partner, to improve relationships
- Increases Fertility, help with Period Cramps and Irregular Periods

What are the Benefits of Full Body Orgasm?

The Human Brain

- Improve body immune system and self-healing mechanism activating Stem cells (via Pineal glands)

- Release of Prolactin to enhance immune system and create a Relaxed state

- Enhance the production of Endorphins (in Pituitary Gland),making people more balanced with their Masculine-Feminine, relaxed, healthy, giving pleasure and happiness reducing tension and stress

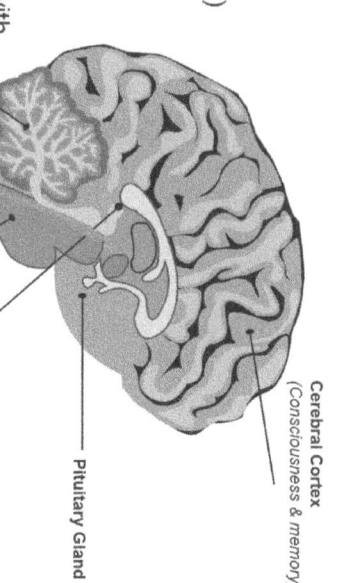

Cerebral Cortex
(Consciousness & memory)

Pituitary Gland

Pineal Gland

Brain Stem

Spinal Cord

Cerebellum
(Muscle Coordination)

Putting Deep Bodywork into Practice

The Deep Bodywork that 1 carry out in a Tantric Journey healing session helps to dissolve negative thoughts, feelings, issues and blocks and will create sufficient positive energies that will spread throughout your body to heal every cell.

This treatment gives the client ultimate control of the pace and focus of the healing. Tantric Journey teaches the body and mind to self-heal, self-develop and to master the skills of achieving a full body, extended Multi Orgasmic Response (MORE), instead of a localized genital release, putting the woman in charge of her own sexuality, instead of depending on a man, woman or even a vibrator.

What to Expect if You Come for Healing

After removing your shoes you will be brought into my Tantric Journey Temple, filled with statues of Buddha, Gods and Goddesses such as Shiva, Shakti, Ganesh and Tara, dim tranquil lighting with candles and incense surrounded with a touch of ethnic ancient music. This is a place of calm and relaxation where there is no agenda or expectations. This is a sacred space to be in, to be fully present and where you will be able to live in your own truth, with no judgment. You may have lived a lie all your life to satisfy your environment, culture, religion, friends, relationships, relatives, work colleagues and neighbours making you totally disconnected to be someone else. It's a place to find yourself, to be connected and it is a time to chat about your massage experiences, expectations, medical history, lifestyle and personal boundaries, likes and dislikes. I will give you a brief history of myself and I am happy to answer any questions you may have. It is paramount for me that you are comfortable and feel at ease with me and the healing you are about to experience.

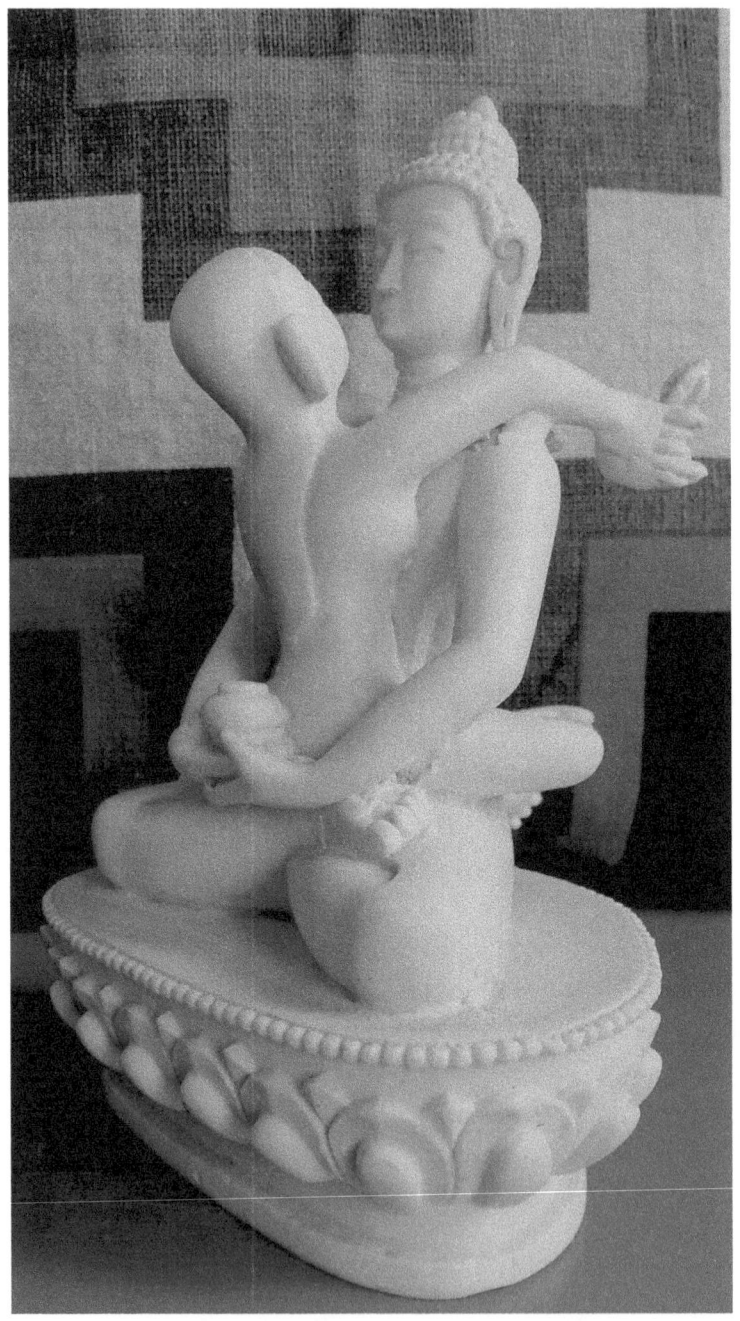

Tantric Journey begins with four key practices:

- Deep breathing with attention
- Movement with feelings
- Chanting with expression of emotions
- Tantric massage to evoke negative imprints

A detailed list of the treatment procedure Treatment Card will be given and a consent form will need to be signed prior to the treatment. Sessions take between three to six hours, depending on the needs of the individual client

Healing Touch

Tantric Journey is not just Tantra work, but instead a unique combination of the following Therapies that I have learned from some of the world famous body workers and healers as follows:

- Charles and Caroline Muir's - Tantra
- Mantak Chia – Tao
- Dr Jack Painter – Deep Bodywork
- Brandon Bay – Journey Therapy
- Aunty Margret – Lomi – Lomi healing massage
- Bodhi Avinasha's – Ipsalu Tantra Cobra breath
- Margot Anand – Osho's white Tantra
- Robert Bay – NLP

My unique learning experience and extensive working practice has led to me developing Tantric Journey that allows me to incorporate my vast wealth of learning and knowledge and includes the following therapies:

1. Holistic Body Therapy
2. Aromatherapy
3. Reflexology
4. Indian Head Massage
5. Hawaiian Lomi-Lomi Massage
6. Swedish Massage
7. Shiatsu
8. Thai Yoga Massage

9. Tantric Healing Massage
10. Pelvic-Heart Integration
11. Lymphatic Drainage Massage
12. Deep Tissue Massage
13. Sacred Spot (Prostate or G-spot) Massage and Yoni Healing
14. Kahuna Healing Massage
15. Emotional and Physical Release Detox Massage
16. Spiritual Hot Rock Massage
17. Journey Therapy
18. Aspects of Counselling
19. Yoga Stretches
20. Breath work and Meditation
21. Toning (with sounds), Mantras and Visualization
22. Cobra breath
23. Tao practices – Chi Nei Tsang (Internal organ – abdominal massage) and Karsai Nei Tsang – (therapeutic genital massage)
24. Life Pulse Massage

After all my learning what I found was that I knew already how to heal people, and we all do. We just need to unblock our emotions that are blocking our true healing potential. What I learnt is that all of us are healers and experts only if we can remove our blocks. This means we don't have to learn any massage modalities to do the healing work I do.

I help my clients reintegrate their Mind and Body connection through a powerful spiritual treatment for awakening and deep healing. The sexual energy within our bodies affects our whole being. I help my clients to recognise how the mind, body, soul, emotions and feelings are all intrinsically linked to each other through the endocrine system, nervous system, circulation and the immune system etc.

There is no disputing that our sexuality can bring us into contact with the most intense of feelings which impact on every level of our presence. When we come to understand how sexual energy flows through us we can learn to harness, support and strengthen it. This energy is vital to us and affects our whole being. It can be spread across the whole body, filling us with health and vitality. When this energy flows it can be used to cultivate health, spiritual growth, creativity and inner peace.

We live in an orgasm-focused society. Orgasm is perceived as being the main achievement in a sexually fulfilled life. In my line of work, it is often perceived that the purpose of the Yoni massage is simply that of achieving the big 'O'. I'm here to tell you it's not. However, I have seen hundreds of clients who feel "broken" because they are unable to achieve the coveted prize of the climax. I have seen many women who feel pressured and distressed by the notion that all 'real' women can orgasm. We are so invested in the notion of orgasms that "faking" orgasms is common; indeed most women admit to having done so at some point in their life.

Despite societies' misguided notion that orgasm is the primary reason to have sex, many women find it impossible and it shouldn't be the primary focus of a fulfilling relationship, but it does perform some very important functions and probably ones that you haven't considered before.

According to several major studies, only 25 percent of women always climax during sex with a partner. The remainder of women either hit or miss — depending on the night, or never experience a female orgasm during intercourse at all. For many women, the female "O" is a fleeting phenomenon.

There are many obstacles that can undermine a woman's capacity to achieve orgasm. I can explain my theory of why some women struggle to achieve orgasm by discussing the function of the orgasm. Orgasm s a positive energy flow that moves from the pelvis to the crown, where the wave of sexual energy activates the pineal glands in the brain to stimulate and connect the nervous system and the endocrine system to send messages to stem cells in every cell in our body. These messages facilitate repair where needed and rejuvenate every cell in our body making us young, healthy and happy. Most people experience their orgasms at a genital level, like a sneeze between the groins, which does not produce a long enough wave to reach the pineal gland and receive benefits from this function.

What is stopping the creation of this long wave and making it travel towards the crown? It is simply our negative emotions, such as fear, shame, sadness etc. as a result of our childhood experiences and upbringing, which stunts the creation of this natural prolonged wave.

During a Tantric Journey session with my female clients, I help them to release both physical and emotional toxins from the body, thus making the body more positively charged. Then I go beyond to facilitate female ejaculation to help them release deeply held negative emotions during a yoni (vaginal) massage.

The Healer as a Catalyst

Features of Bodywork

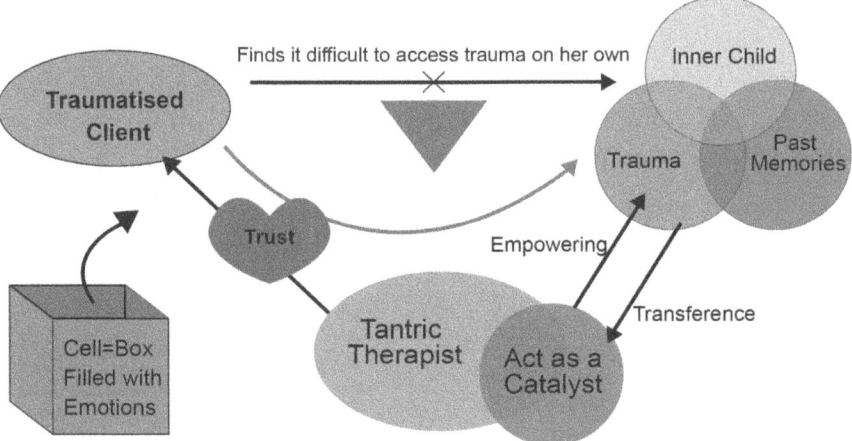

During my years as a tantric healer I have learned that it's not the therapist who heals the client during Deep Bodywork, but it's the client who heals herself, in the presence of a trusting therapist who can hold the space to enable the woman to release emotions freely. The therapist only acts as a catalyst to help the client access stagnant negative imprints as a result of past trauma (rather than accessing old trauma by herself) by working on trigger points where the trauma is stored.

Once the emotions are fully felt in the client's body, it's a certain deep breathing technique that enables her to release and unblock the stagnant negative emotions. She may feel fear, sadness, anger etc., during the treatment as a result of Deep Bodywork. The time it can go wrong is due to lack of understanding of our own bodies and emotions. It's important to note that sometimes transference and projections can take place, which means that the clients will blame the therapist for the way they feel. This is the danger that all good massage therapists may experience, which is why we need to take special care in dealing with women who have experienced trauma.

During my therapy sessions, I often introduce a client's partner into the process by helping him learn to communicate and connect with his partner. One of the biggest obstacles to this process is that my male clients often feel threatened or uncomfortable with the idea of getting in touch with their "feminine" side in order to enhance communication with their partner.

What's stopping the man from becoming feminine is that he's blocking his negative emotions, just like a woman. He's blocking his negative emotions in the feminine body. And these negative emotions are stored the same as in the woman. Women's deepest negative emotions are stored in the female prostate or in the G-spot, whilst in the man, feminine emotions are stored in the male prostate. So if you can do the Bodywork on the man and massage the male prostate regularly, you can get in touch with the feminine side of the man; that means he will become more feminine and balanced.

It's important to reassure male clients that balancing male and female energies is nothing to do with sexual orientation nor is it connected to losing being balanced with the masculine and the feminine energy. One of the biggest problems we have in society at the moment is that men are too masculine and macho, and they are not connected to their feminine side of the body. That's why they can't understand and communicate with women.

If a man wants to get in touch with his feminine side, he needs to go to a female Tantric Journey Healer in order to preserve the yin-yang equilibrium. She will do exactly the work I do with a woman, for example the male prostate massage with breathing exercises, movements, and vocal sounds. It's likely that he will cry, get angry, and release emotions – and that's when he's become in touch with his feminine side of the body. That's when he'll become much more balanced as a result of his equal masculine and feminine energies. He would be a much better lover for a woman than a masculine man, as he would be capable of getting in touch with her heart centre before he contacts her sex centre.

At the same time, the woman who is receiving the Yoni massage and releasing negative emotions gets in touch with the masculine side of the body. For example, men are not scared to get a massage or to have the lingam massage. They are not shy, they don't feel sad, and they don't cry, but that's the masculine side of the body. So when a woman releases all the negatives energies in her body, she will be able to get in touch with the masculine side of the body and then men will love that masculine side of her body which is now more open and connected with the sex centre. This aids connection and allows the woman to get in touch with her own goddess and be more balanced.

A relationship can function much better when each person can get in touch with the opposite polarities. They're able to communicate with one another, understand each other's emotions and motivations, and help each other become more enlightened human beings. It's the completion of the yin-yang balance; when this has been achieved, the relationship can become more fulfilling, positive, and sensual.

Many men are still afraid to undergo the healing powers of the Tantric Journey. They think that it somehow makes them effeminate or less of a man. To them, I say this: every man is made up of masculine and feminine energies (masculine and feminine hormones). A person who is only in touch with his masculine side is only half a man. Being a stunted human means that you'll live a stunted life – that's why it's so important for men to put aside this ultra-macho attitude, because it's only infusing their bodies with negative, poisonous energies.

The Male G-Spot (Prostate)

Male and female G-spots have more in common than one might think; in fact, there's nothing different between the female G-spot and the male G-spot (the prostate). Both have the same functions, although the medical community is still grappling with what purposes those functions might serve. But for the purposes of Tantric Journey healing, the G-spot is akin to a storehouse of emotions. This is the place where men store their negative energies; in fact, I estimate that about 80% of negative emotions are stored within the prostate, while the rest of the body holds 20% of the emotions. This is why Tantric Journey healing for men focuses on massaging the prostate, because like the yoni, this is where the negative energies are the most focused. With this respect, the G-spot isn't even related to sexuality; in fact, I like to tell the story about one client who suddenly evoked the memory of her two year old brother dying when I was massaging her G-spot. Now this brother has nothing to do with her sexually but it's the sadness that she had because of the brother dying. The G-spot is a powerful holder of negative emotions, which is why it plays a central role in the Tantric Journey healing process.

My Estimate

20% Problem and Solution = In the Body
80% Problem and Solution = In the Prostate

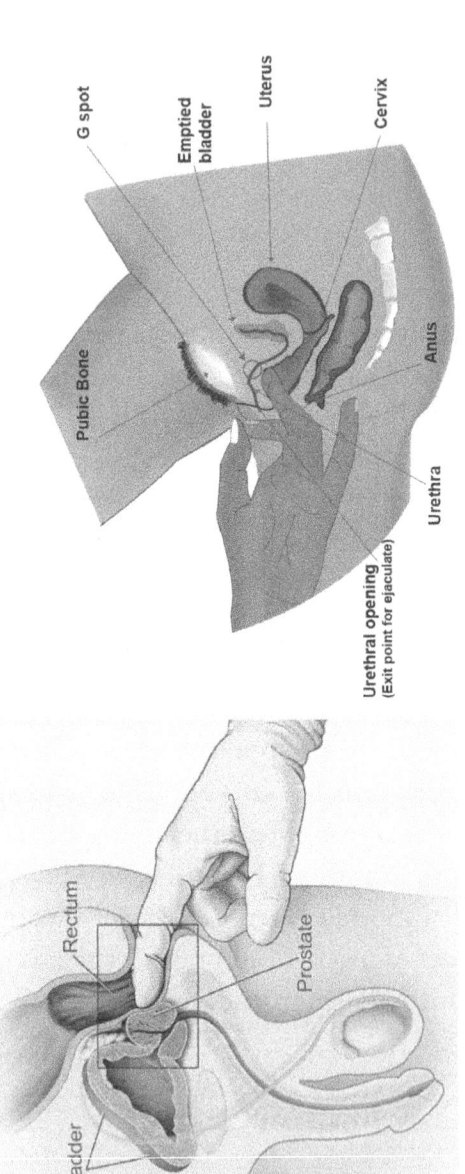

Female Prostate (G-Spot)

Male Prostate(G-Spot)

As previously mentioned, if a man wants to undergo Tantric Journey healing, he needs to see a female healer. She can help him release the frustrations, sadness and anger that has been building up in his G-spot, which is often why men want sex so quickly that they're willing to go to a prostitute to pay for the release of the pressure that they build up due to stagnate emotions in the male prostate, which puts pressure to ejaculate to release the sexual tension. He wants to ejaculate because essentially he wants to release the tension without having to deal with the emotions he is experiencing, whereas a woman will suppress the emotions in the body rather than exploring the sexual release feelings he's experiencing, whereas a woman doesn't usually have that opportunity or drive. A man isn't usually conscious of this need; he's stagnant with negative emotions and he's looking to relieve the tension by ejaculating quickly. That's often why rape and abuse occur, because a man is urgently looking for a way to release his tension. He's thinking at the time that he's doing her a favour; that's his unconscious way of making love to her.

So now if he can get his prostrate massaged and release negative emotions from this pent-up place, the man will be able to experience positive feelings that will last. He will no longer need to feel as though he must ejaculate quickly, because he'll always be able to ejaculate when he wants. That's because there's no more negative emotion that's putting the pressure on his prostate.

If the prostate is healthy and if there is no negative emotions, there's a lot of positive emotions. Then the male client can learn to separate the orgasm from the ejaculation. Once you learn to separate the orgasm and the ejaculation, that's when you can effectively make love to a woman. Women take a long time to orgasm, whilst men only take a few minutes. If a man wants to actually make love to a woman and to give her an orgasm, then the man must learn how to withhold the ejaculation and stay with the woman as long as she takes. Because otherwise, what happens in every relationship, is that the man ejaculates so quickly that he just goes to sleep once he's finished. Meanwhile the woman is wondering what just happened.

Orgasmic wave of a Happy Couple

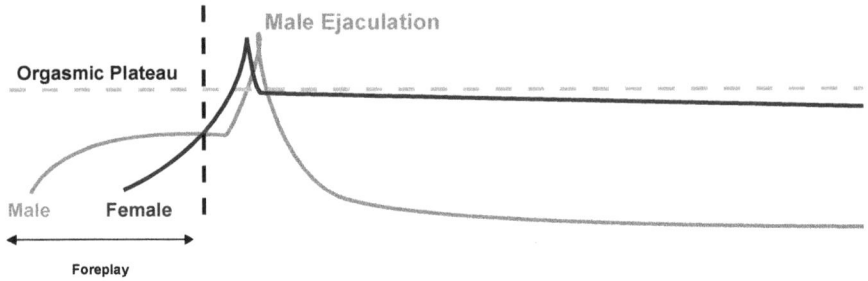

Comparison of the Arousal Pattern of Men versus Women

Sometimes the man will think he has so much to prove (this is male ego as a result of a blocked prostate) that he goes in too quickly, which ends up being incredibly painful for the woman; this is why she fakes an orgasm to stop him, because she doesn't know how to tell him, "You're a bad lover". She doesn't want to damage his ego; she just wants the sex to stop. She loves him too much to damage his ego. But what becomes damaging is when this goes on every time.

If a man gets in touch with his feminine side, however, he'll begin to keep up with his lover so that they both can enjoy the positive relief that comes from a full-body orgasm. What's more, he can learn how to have hundreds of orgasms without even ejaculating and that makes him a much better lover and partner. Believe me, that's enough of a motivator to get a man to undergo much needed Tantric healing!

Massaging the prostate can also help treat one of the biggest killers of men: prostate cancer. When negative emotions accumulate within the prostate, this means that healthy blood circulation is being blocked from the sexual organs. If you think of a tube - like a hose pipe - and it's blocked inside, then the water can't go at the same speed. Capillaries are so small and only one blood cell can go through this tiny tube. So imagine that if you have got even the tiniest block in the capillaries, then you'll have a reduced blood flow going into the sexual organs or any other organ.

This not only means that it's harder for men to become aroused, but it also prevents the prostate from functioning properly. When the prostate is regularly massaged, it can help clear up the blockages and release the toxins that can lead to prostate cancer. And this is serious for men's health; after all, hundreds of thousands of men die from prostate cancer every year. By undergoing regular prostate massages, you can help ensure that blood flow is being properly managed, thus protecting your overall health.

But it's important to note that massage will only help to release the negative emotions in the body; you need to go on an actual detox to remove any physical toxicity in the body. What you eat and drink can contribute to the blockages within your prostate. Therefore, a man's ideal health can be achieved through a combination of good diet, exercise, and regular prostate massages that will release both the emotional toxins and the physical toxins.

Self-Discipline for the Man

When a client comes to me the first thing I do is meet her exactly where she is, emotionally, at that time. Even to arrive for the first session, she often has to overcome some of the strongest barriers of shame, fear, and guilt or mistrust, which may have been with her for many years. I accept all the barriers and fears, without forcing any change. I understand that the outcome she wants from a treatment is to be free from her issues, but this must be approached with the greatest sensitivity and respect for her emotions. Full unconditional acceptance is key to developing trust.

We may take a long time in Talking therapy sessions before any Bodywork can be done, which also helps to develop connection, trust, and open the mind for treatment. Clients may have questions, or a lack of knowledge about the treatment or their own issues, which can be fully explained through dialogue, including preparing her for what can actually happen during a treatment.

When we begin Bodywork, it is fully clothed, using Tantric Journey Level 1 (Thai-Yoga massage) techniques. This is a safe and comfortable place for most women to start, and helps to further develop trust while being in itself a powerful treatment. When she is completely comfortable and ready, we can go on to massaging partly uncovered areas of body, and when the time is right we can massage fully naked using Tantric Journey Level 2 techniques. This process of uncovering the body is often mirrored in the experience of uncovering emotions. By the time a woman feels comfortable enough to be naked she is more ready to open to deeper healing. It is like peeling an onion. Each layer of clothing represents an emotion. The top layer can be shame or fear and so forth.

After a few sessions of deep full body massages, and once she is comfortably opening physically, emotionally and energetically, I can then introduce the Yoni Healing massage using Tantric Journey massage techniques. During the yoni (vaginal) massage it is important, as in all aspects of treatment, not to force any outcome, especially ejaculation. Ejaculation requires a very deep level of trust and for the body to totally surrender.

For me as a practitioner, there are important basic principles which always guide my work. One is that my client is always right, and that it is imperative that I hold the space unconditionally and without judgment for her to acknowledge and express her emotions fully. There are no right or wrong emotions and in order for emotions to flow and be released we must fully welcome them all.

Another is that a woman can always change her mind at any time, as emotions behave much like waves in the sea; sometimes approaching, sometimes receding, sometimes washing over and through us. They are constantly changing, both positive and negative. This must be respected fully. The woman is always in control, and it is my job to be her student and learn fast. She is totally individual in her needs and desires in any moment, and it is important that I drop my ego and my own ideas about how a session proceeds and comply with what she wants and needs at all times.

Finally, to work always with unconditional love, and to treat all women equally knowing that every woman is different, and the same woman is different in every moment. It can be magical to watch a client open and expand her experience with the support and safe space I can provide. Indeed it is an honour to be able to accompany a woman on her journey of self-discovery and healing.

Orgasm vs. Ejaculation for Men

There seems to be a common belief that a man can't orgasm without ejaculating. As I've mentioned before throughout this book, this is a false belief, as men can learn to orgasm without ever ejaculating. Taking the Tantric Journey can allow men to enjoy all the pleasures of the orgasm, as he will learn how to control the ejaculation process.

When men take the Tantric Journey, it allows them to go through the process of emotional release. When men feel an incessant urge to ejaculate, this is because their negative emotions are creating a blockage in the prostate, which is building up a sense of tension and urgency within the body. Men tend to ejaculate quickly when they're experiencing this tension, only to have it build up again. This is because they're only relieving the symptoms, not the actual problem. If a man wants to learn how to have an orgasm without actually ejaculating, he needs to go through the process of emotional release to get to that stage. Similar to the Yoni massage, this involves a deep, but gentle massage of the prostate, which allows the negative energies to be released.

Male Prostate (Male G – spot)

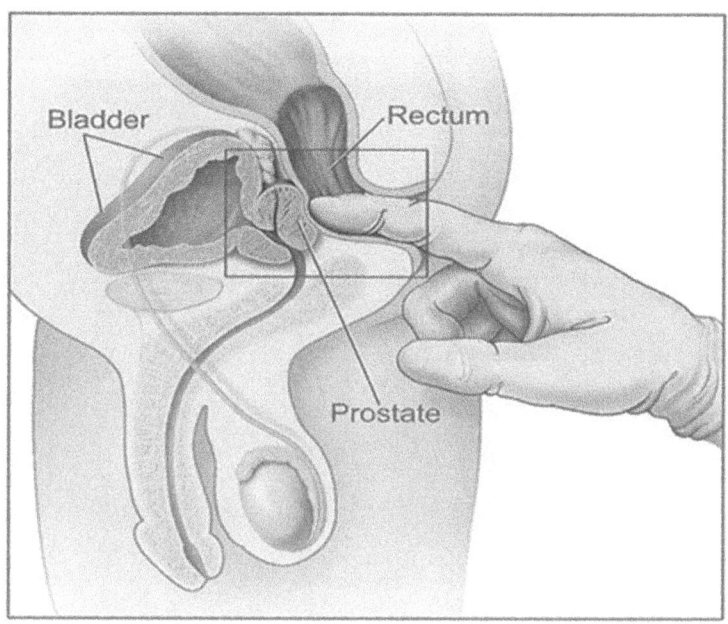

The Tantric Journey allows the man to understand what pleasure points he needs to get to before he must hold himself back from ejaculating. Think about it in terms of masturbation, with a numerical scale reflecting the amount of pleasure that the man is experiencing. If 10 represents the point where the man is about to ejaculate, 9 is the point of no return while 8 is the point just before point of no return. This is the point where masturbation of the lingam must stop and draw the sexual energy inwards with deep breathing without ejaculating outwards. Each shot of male ejaculation consist of approximately 300 – 400 million sperms, which can populate Europe. So you can imagine how much energy is used with one ejaculation alone. When this ejaculation is withheld and moved inwards into the body it produces equal amount of benefits to the body.

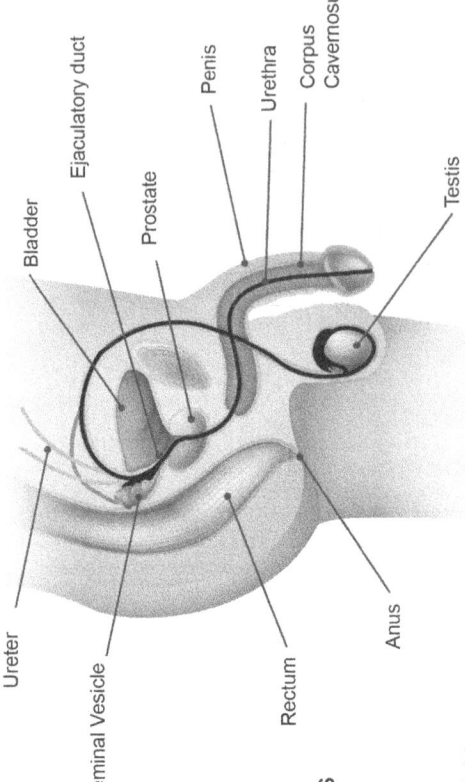

- Bladder
- Ejaculatory duct
- Prostate
- Penis
- Urethra
- Corpus Cavernosum
- Testis
- Ureter
- Seminal Vesicle
- Rectum
- Anus

Male Ejaculation

- Each ejaculation has 300 - 400 million sperms

- Each sperm consists of "Energy"

- One male ejaculation can populate entire Europe

- This is the amount loss of energy for a man with one ejaculation

- This is the reason why men go to sleep and get tired after an orgasm with ejaculation

- Regular ejaculation will reduce his lifespan

This means that millions of sperm energy is moving around, creating a great deal of energy and a sense of renewal within the body. Sperm is an incredible harnesser of energy, which is why the man should be brought to the brink of that seven or eight times. Eventually, the man's erection will go down, and this is where he'll experience the amazing energy that comes from having millions of sperm energy moving around his chakra from pelvic basin to crown. He hasn't ejaculated this energy; instead, he's harnessing it as a positive and powerful force. The man will feel the pleasure, longevity, empowerment and electric energy that comes from having orgasms without the ejaculation. That means he can make love to his partner as long as she needs, thus being able to give her multiple orgasms.

When a man has gone on a Tantric Journey he can learn the art of conscious loving, not having to do much with the ego, but to make love in stillness. He'll be able to control his ejaculation, which means he can make love to his partner over and over again. Women can take hours to reach the point of ejaculation and or orgasm; when a man takes the Tantric Journey, he can make love with her for whatever amount of time she needs in order to facilitate her orgasm.

This technique also has really positive effects on fertility for although men produce millions of sperm a day (compared to the 300–400 eggs that women release during their lifetime), because sperm cells take about seventy-five days to grow to maturity, harming them can affect your fertility and frequent ejaculation reduces the chances of conception and your own life span.

A man who is able to preserve and cultivate this sexual energy is like a honeypot to women. They are able to sense when a man is filled with this positive and sexual energy, which is why they'll be irresistibly drawn to him. This is how men can empower themselves; they'll have the sexual energy to ensure that they're always attracting a woman with equally positive energy, or keeping the family together with the positive energy and sexuality that the woman will always be drawn to.

What's more, learning how to harness this sexual energy makes it easier for men to look and feel younger. When I talked about the yoni massage, I mentioned that women just look younger as soon as they experience female ejaculation. The same goes for men; once they learn how to withhold ejaculation so they can please their lovers, they'll look 10, maybe even 20 years younger than before. It's really an incredible result that more men should know about – in fact, I like to joke that the Tantric Journey is better than any anti-wrinkle cream or surgical operation!

Keeping Up with a Woman

One of the biggest problems that men have when they're making love to a woman is that they don't know how to keep up with her. The man doesn't need the amount of time the woman does in order to reach orgasm; that's why you find that the man is ready to orgasm and fall asleep, while the woman is left wondering, "What about me?"

This is where the problem is in many relationships. That's why the man has to learn how to withhold his ejaculation so that he can be just as empowered as the woman. Men don't understand that it's possible to separate the orgasm from ejaculation. If the man knows how to separate the orgasm and the ejaculation, then he can have lots of orgasms with his partner without ever having to ejaculate.

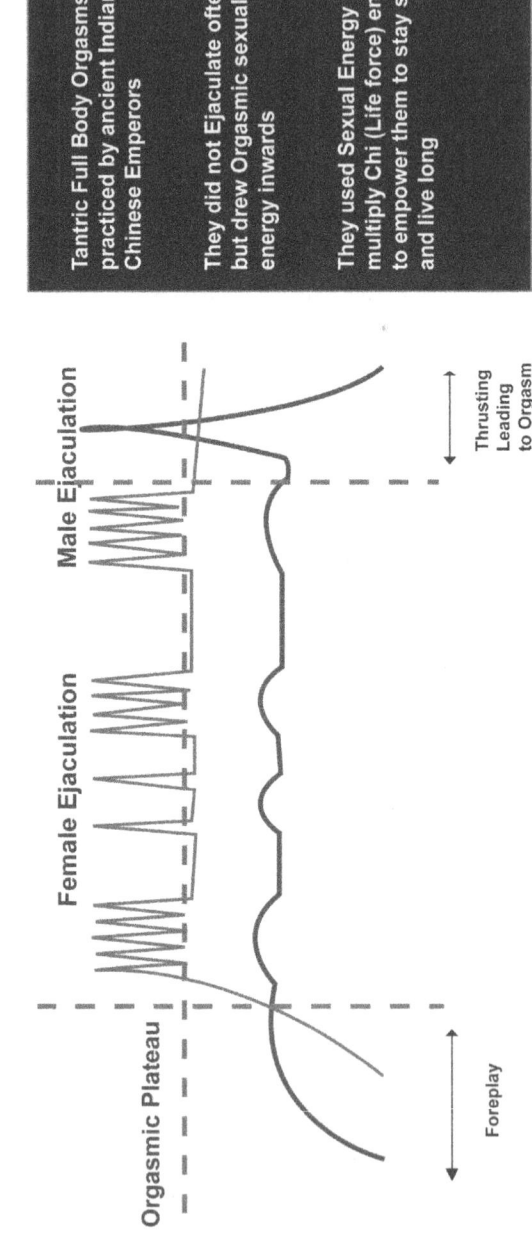

Orgasmic wave of a Tantric Couple

Tantric Full Body Orgasms were practiced by ancient Indian and Chinese Emperors

They did not Ejaculate often but drew Orgasmic sexual energy inwards

They used Sexual Energy to multiply Chi (Life force) energy to empower them to stay strong and live long

Male Ejaculation

Female Ejaculation

Orgasmic Plateau

Thrusting Leading to Orgasm

Foreplay

The Multiple Orgasms Pattern of Women

Men learn how to do this by visiting a female Tantric Journey therapist, who can perform a lingam, testicle and prostate massage. When the man feels as though he's about to ejaculate, she has to stop the man and engage in breathing exercises. During this time, she'll start massaging the head, neck, and shoulders so that she can draw the energy that she created in the lingam upward. When you do this ten or twenty times, the lingam gets trained how to withhold ejaculation and draw the energy toward the body through breathing. This means he'll know how to stop before he ejaculates so he can draw all of that energy into his mind. The purpose of the simultaneous prostate massage is to dissolve the negative stagnate emotions in the male prostate.

This energy is a result of over 300 – 400 million sperm, which means he'll have life force energy humming throughout his body. Being filled with this kind of sexual energy is very healing, because it fills his entire body with the kind of warm, positive energy that flushes out all the negative emotions and trauma that may be trapped within his cellular memory.

This is perhaps the best treatment for men who not only need emotional healing, but also have difficulties with erections and premature ejaculation. All of these problems can be boiled down to emotional issues that are within the man's body; therefore, when he engages in these breathing exercises, he'll be able to release and overcome the negative energies and emotions that are preventing him from satisfying his lover, because he'll be able to separate his orgasm from his ejaculation.

Men often have trouble remembering that in order to make love, you don't necessarily need an erection. Men often get caught up in this line of thinking because they believe they need to have a rock-hard erection just to satisfy a woman, but this is a false belief that's perpetuated by pornography and overtly sexualized cultural beliefs. A man who is focusing on his erection doesn't realise that women can also be aroused by relaxing the mind and body, which can often be done through the art of the healing massage. Sometimes men get so focused looking for sex that they don't realize women aren't always looking for the same level of physicality as they are. Men who can't get erections can still be fantastic lovers, as long as they know how to utilise that sexual energy from the lingam to transfer it throughout the entire body.

Awakening the Woman

As I explained earlier, women get aroused through the relaxation of the mind and body. So to relax her mind, the man must do everything positive to understand and accept the woman for who she is and where she is emotionally. He needs to understand that her emotions are changing all the time. He needs to take time and to listen in order to fully gain her trust. He must be sincere and genuine in his intentions and in what he tells her otherwise he will damage the connection.

Once the woman's mind is relaxed, the man needs to relax the woman's body by massaging her shoulders. A woman holds a lot of tension within her shoulders, so it's important for a man to massage the shoulders before having sex. He can also do a nice, firm massage around the head, neck, lower back, the buttocks, and even the calves. If he does this for about 10 to 15 minutes, her body will begin to relax – but that's only if he's going at the right speed. All this touch must be done with firmness but slowly and with no expectations.

Men might want to quickly go through the massage in order to get to the sex, but that's not what the woman wants. If he touches the woman at half speed or at stillness, she'll experience the kind of arousal that's needed for intimate lovemaking.

Once the man matches the woman's energy with a slower massage, she'll begin to open up, breathe a little more deeply, and she'll begin to move around from becoming aroused. It's important for the man to ignore all of these invitations, because it's still too early to have sex. He should continue to carry on with a slow and deep massage for about 15 to 20 minutes so that the body will just melt like butter. Whatever problems she was having will just be gone, which will help the woman to become even more aroused.

How to Win and Keep a Woman's Love

There are a few golden rules for men to follow in order to win a woman's love and lifelong companionship.

- Always say "I understand how you feel" when she is emotional and mean it when you say it
- Make her believe that she is always right, even when you know in your logical mind that she is wrong
- Accept her when she changes her mind any time she wants
- Don't blame her; don't try to fix her. Accept who she is in the moment without judgment
- Love her with no expectations
- Keep your doors open, to let her share everything with you. Man becomes the vessel for her to download all her emotions as and when she needs and you must listen but not react. This will be very difficult to do for a man with extreme masculine energy with a high ego, but easy to do with a man who has got in touch with his feminine energy to be a balanced man.

Yoni Massage

The yoni massage is no different than the massage of any other part of the body. However, it's important for a man to realise that he has to do the massage very slowly, as doing it quickly will cause a woman to shut down. During the yoni massage, try not to stimulate the clitoris too much, as you want to ensure that this orgasm is coming from the G-spot rather than from the clitoris, which is similar to a penis orgasm. We're not trying to put her to sleep with a clitoral orgasm; we're trying to awaken her. While doing the yoni massage, perform the G-spot massage and the A-spot massage; the A-spot is just below the cervix, and it gives her even deeper pleasure than a G-spot massage.

Yoni (Vaginal) Spots Of A Woman
(Reservoirs that hold emotions)

The U - Spot

This is a small patch of sensitive erectile tissue *located just above and on either side of the urethral opening*. It is absent just below the urethra. In the small area between the urethra and the vagina

The G - Spot

This is a small, highly sensitive area located 5-8 cm *(2-3 inches)* *inside the vagina*. On the front or upper wall

The A - Spot

Its true location is *just above the cervix, at the innermost point of the vagina*. The cervix of the uterus is the narrow part that protrudes slightly into the vagina, leaving a circular recess around itself.

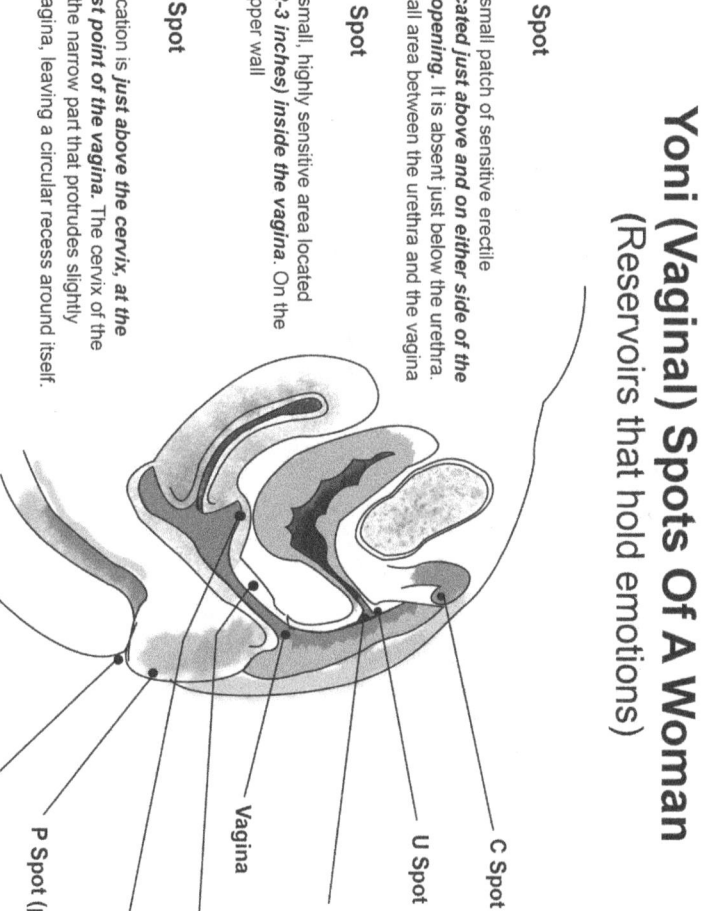

C Spot (Clitoris)

U Spot

Urethra

Vagina

G Spot

A Spot

P Spot (perineum)

Anus

Yoni (Vaginal) Spots Of A Woman
(Reservoirs that hold emotions)

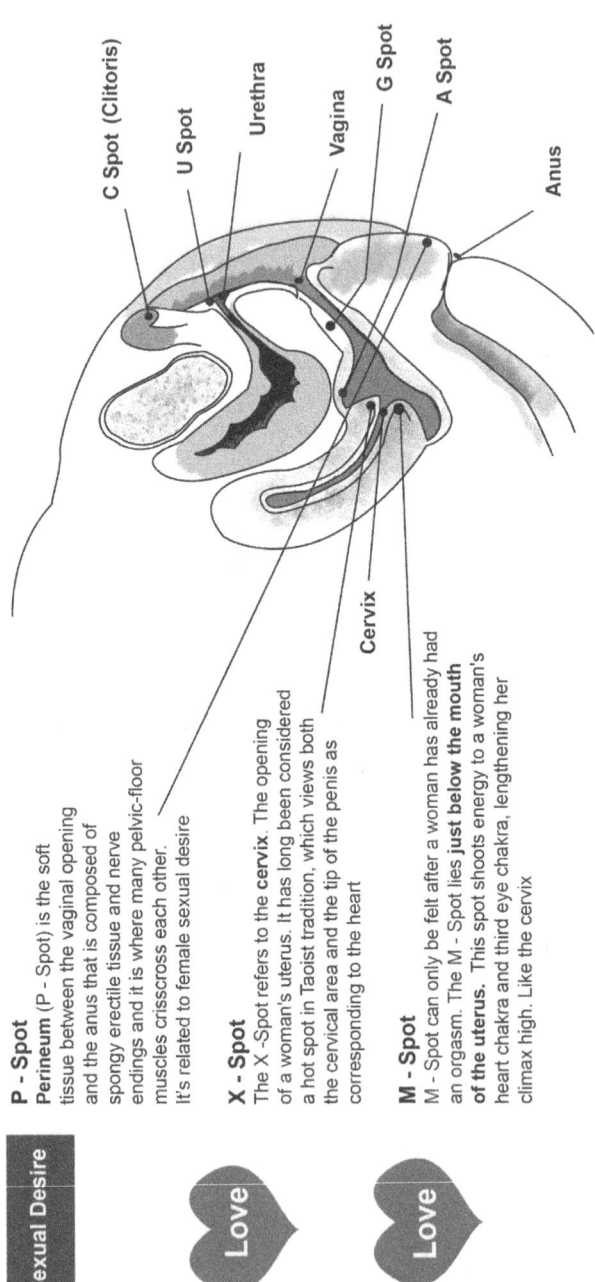

C Spot (Clitoris)

U Spot

Urethra

Vagina

G Spot

A Spot

Anus

Cervix

Sexual Desire

Love

Love

P - Spot
Perineum (P - Spot) is the soft tissue between the vaginal opening and the anus that is composed of spongy erectile tissue and nerve endings and it is where many pelvic-floor muscles crisscross each other. It's related to female sexual desire

X - Spot
The X -Spot refers to the **cervix**. The opening of a woman's uterus. It has long been considered a hot spot in Taoist tradition, which views both the cervical area and the tip of the penis as corresponding to the heart

M - Spot
M - Spot can only be felt after a woman has already had an orgasm. The M - Spot lies **just below the mouth of the uterus.** This spot shoots energy to a woman's heart chakra and third eye chakra, lengthening her climax high. Like the cervix

If the woman asks the man to make love to her, he still needs to ignore this request, because he needs to focus on the yoni massage. She'll continue to breathe deeply, make a lot of sounds and move her body, which means she's building desire. Only when the woman has asked you three times throughout the yoni massage should you start making love to her. If the man doesn't have an erection at this point, it's not a problem; you can penetrate without having an erection. All he needs to do is to go inside of her, and she'll need to squeeze her pelvic muscles around him so that she's massaging the lingam. When she does this, she's actually massaging the lingam so that it slowly awakens. For a woman to be able to successfully massage the lingam with the vaginal muscles, she needs to strengthen her vaginal muscles with 'sexercises' discussed in the following chapter. Once she strengthens each ring of the vaginal muscles, she will be able to use the vagina like a flute to create rhythmic waves in the Yoni to massage the lingam.

Strengthening the Pelvic Floor

It's important for the woman to learn how to strengthen her pelvic floor muscles by exercising her Pubococcygeus muscles (PC muscles) a hundred to two hundred times each and every day. When she squeezes the muscles, she breathes through the nose; when she relaxes she breathes out through the mouth. She needs to do this process every day for about three to six months to strengthen her yoni muscles so that she can massage the lingam with the yoni. That way, the man won't feel pressured to get an erection before entering, because she can just use her PC muscles to massage and awaken the lingam when it's inside her. The yoni will also be able to create sexual energy even when a man is unable to gain an erection.

One way to help a woman strengthen her PC muscles is to use the jade egg, which can be inserted into the yoni. Jade eggs have a natural high vibration. The Chinese have always valued jade because of its balanced yin-yang energy. The Jade Egg "sexercises" provide more power to the Chi Muscle to lift the sexual energy inward and upward, where it can be circulated to the other vital organs and help to balance the monthly flow of blood and daily cycle of hormones, thus improving, the vital energy and overall well-being of the woman.

The sexercises strengthen and control the Chi Muscle. It is easier to practice control of this muscle with a jade egg inside the vagina since, as the egg moves, you can feel the direction in which the Chi Muscle moves.

Jade Egg to Strengthen the Pelvic Floor Muscles

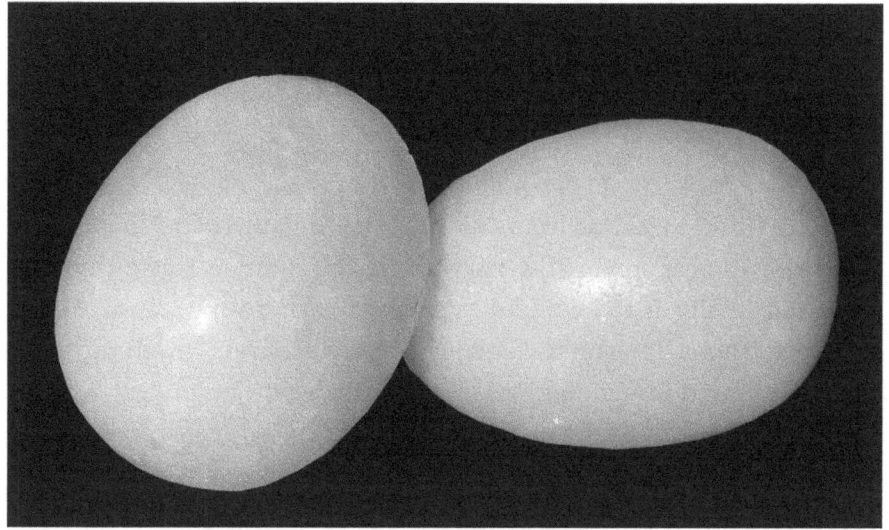

Let Women Create the Rhythm

When making love, it is important for the lingam to stay in stillness until the woman creates the rhythm; if the man creates a rhythm, it's too difficult for the woman to follow his rhythm because it's too overpowering. If a woman creates her own sexual rhythm, she'll become aroused in her own way. This is the best way she can become aroused and open up, as the man's rhythm will only cause her to shut down. Then it becomes very difficult for her to start again, so she'll probably just fake an orgasm just for the man to stop quickly. If a man really loves a woman, he'll make every effort to follow her rhythm to help her awaken. Once she's reached this point, he won't even have to do anything, because everything will be done by the woman.

As you can see, it's very easy to make a woman orgasmic, but you need to learn these little techniques first. Being a good lover means you're not just focused on your own physical pleasure; you're focused on the woman's pleasure as well. You need to make lovemaking a safe place for your woman, instead of letting ego take over so that you're just focused on ejaculating as soon as possible.

Male Exercise to Prolong Release

When a man enters a woman, he should only enter with the lingam head, at the entrance of the yoni. The man does not even need to have an erection. In this position, thrusting can only be done at the entrance; he should thrust nine times, and at the tenth thrust, he should go deep inside and thrust once more. After the tenth thrust, he should go back to the entrance of the yoni, and thrust eight times; on the ninth thrust, he should go back deep inside the yoni to thrust twice. He should continue to count down like this, because it will occupy the man's mind so that he's not thinking of ejaculating; he's just focused on these numbers. The thrusting must be done very slowly. The slower the thrusting the more arousing it is to the woman.

He's actually going into a deep state of meditation, which is one way that he can control his desires to ejaculate as soon as possible. This also helps the two partners find the woman's rhythm, which is where the real sexual arousal will start building and peaking to multiple orgasms.

So to summaries the 10 counts are as follows, with very slow movements with stillness at the end of each round:

9 shallow thrusts with 1 deep thrust
8 shallow thrusts with 2 deep thrusts
7 shallow thrusts with 3 deep thrusts

6 shallow thrusts with 4 deep thrusts
5 shallow thrusts with 5 deep thrusts
4 shallow thrusts with 6 deep thrusts
3 shallow thrusts with 7 deep thrusts
2 shallow thrusts with 8 deep thrusts
1 shallow thrust with 9 deep thrusts

Healthy Male Ejaculation

It's very important to a man to ejaculate from time to time because if he doesn't ejaculate, it puts pressure on his prostate and then that could give him problems as well. The man has to ejaculate into a certain equation. Let's say the man is 50 years old; you divide his age by five, which means he needs to ejaculate every ten days. If the man is 20 years, then divide it by five, he needs to ejaculate every four days. Younger people can ejaculate more frequently, whereas older people need to ejaculate with a longer time elapse. All of this is to preserve the man's life force energy because every time he ejaculates, he loses part of his life. When a man ejaculates, he is releasing his vital essence which is carried out of his body by the semen. From a Taoist perspective, the sperm carry the man's Jing (Primordial Energy) or sexual essence. By going on the Tantric Journey, the man can live longer, look younger, and be happier. This is a huge attraction for women, because they can practically see that sexual energy radiating from the man.

Even a single man can engage in these practices; he just needs to learn how to take himself to the brink of orgasm several times without actually ejaculating. This will build up the life force energy within him, which is very attractive to women, even if you don't look like a Hollywood movie star.

Awakening: female sexuality

Some people are always confounded by the fact that the most beautiful people in the world can still be single. This isn't because there's anything wrong with them; it's because their sexual energies are dormant. Women need to learn how to ejaculate at the same time they have an orgasm, as female ejaculation is important for releasing negative energy from the body via the yoni.

When a woman is filled with positive energy, she'll be in a better place to attract a more positive partner, because she'll be filled with a positive, radiating energy that people just want to be around. As a woman, when you learn how to ejaculate, the orgasms automatically manifest and you won't have to do anything to achieve it.

Self-Healing Mechanisms

The purpose of an orgasm is to heal the body and mind; it can give the body the energy it needs to start repairing and renewing cells. So if a simple orgasm can do this, imagine what healing powers sexual energy can have on your entire body when it's constantly coursing through every cell in your body. Orgasmic energy will be within your head, which is when the real healing begins. This is why it's so important for women to undergo the Tantric Journey if they've experienced a sexual trauma or are filled with negative energy, because it ensures that this sexual energy is helping them to heal. They can start having healthy relationships with men again, and feel pleasure without bringing the trauma into mind. This can also heal a majority of relationship issues, because it opens up the pathways to better communication and lovemaking.

You don't need to go to counselling. If you rid yourself of the problems that are following you, you may not need to go to counselling or psychotherapy and you may not have to keep searching for a new partner. The real answer is to learn how to open up the lines of communication, which can only happen when your entire body is fused with this wonderful sexual energy.

Orgasm and Ejaculation in Women

In my professional experience I have listened to many women and found that a large majority of women have difficulty attaining orgasm. According to statistics, as many as one in three women have trouble reaching orgasm when having sex; as many as 75% percent of women have difficulty achieving orgasm from vaginal intercourse alone. This is not only caused by a man's inability to keep up with the woman's need for hours of foreplay and lovemaking; it's also been popularised by today's society. It is a general trend that there is deemed something wrong with a woman if she doesn't orgasm quickly after penetration, but the nature of a woman means that it can take an hour or more for this state to be reached.

So much emphasis is placed upon the 'need' for achieving a female orgasm, but generally few women and even fewer men know what actually happens when a woman orgasms. That warm rush a woman feels during foreplay is the result of blood heading straight to the vagina and clitoris. Around this time, the walls of the vagina start to secrete beads of lubrication that eventually get bigger and flow together. As you become more turned on, blood continues to flood the pelvic area, breathing speeds up, heart rate increases, nipples become erect, and the lower part of the vagina narrows in order to grip the lingam (penis) while the upper part expands to give it somewhere to go. If the correct emotional and physical stimulation is received, an incredible amount of nerve and muscle tension builds up in the genitals, pelvis, buttocks, and thighs — until the female body involuntarily releases it all at once in a series of intensely pleasurable waves, known as the orgasm.

The big 'o' is the moment when the uterus, vagina, and anus contract simultaneously at 0.8-second intervals. A small orgasm may consist of three to five contractions; whereas an orgasm can consist of 10 to 15. An orgasm is not just about the body though and a recent small-scale study at the Netherlands' University of Groningen found that areas of the brain involving fear and emotion are actually deactivated during orgasm.

An over sexualised culture has led to a false reality for women. The Tantric Journey allows them to realise that they too should play an active role in lovemaking; in fact, they should be the centre of it.

Female ejaculation is the secretion of a clear fluid by a woman during sexual arousal, which can occur at the acme of an orgasm. There are many colloquialisms for this including squirting.

There are no set rules as to the amount of secretion a woman can ejaculate. A woman can release as little as a teaspoonful or a cupful, yet some claim to ejaculate a great deal more than that and I have seen great variances in clients.

Not every woman can easily ejaculate, so don't be disheartened if you've not experienced this. However, every woman has the biological anatomy to ejaculate so it is possible and it is nothing to feel ashamed about.

Female ejaculation has resulted in embarrassment and anguish for many women who have been victims of misinformation. Many women lead their lives unaware of the purpose of the female ejaculation and this lack of knowledge leads to sexual suppression and inability to seek professional help. Ignorance from mainstream medicine has also led to the extremes of surgery and of the trauma that goes with it.

Whilst female ejaculation isn't a myth, it can be an elusive phenomenon for many women because it is not widely or often discussed. In fact, many women feel embarrassed when it happens and think they've urinated on their partner or the bed. Until relatively recently, the medical community didn't even recognise female ejaculation.

As late as the 1980s, many doctors who were aware of the phenomenon of women ejaculating assumed the fluid must be urine, but urine is not the same as female ejaculation. If the medical profession haven't been recognising this vital part of female sexuality in modern history, then it is hardly surprising that it is still largely thought of as a myth.

Thankfully times are changing and an increasing number of medical researchers have come to understand that the liquid comes from the Skene's glands (also known as **vestibular glands, periurethral glands, paraurethral glands**, or female **prostate, G-spot)** which are located on the anterior wall of the vagina around the lower end of the urethra and that the liquid is not that of urine, however, the function of ejaculation is still widely unexplored in mainstream medicine.

The current growth of awareness of this phenomenon has ironically kindled thoughts of inadequacy in some women who do not ejaculate. The reason some women cannot ejaculate is down to blocked negative emotions. The porn industry gives men and women a false representation of the female and of the female ejaculation; whilst people use porn films as a guideline to their love-making, men and women will continue to feel inadequate. Sex should occur without a goal and it must be appreciated that a female orgasm is an implosion unlike the male orgasm that is an explosion.

There is another form of female ejaculation that comes from the A-spot. This is located just on either side of the cervix just above. If you make your index finger and the middle finger, insert them into the yoni and open the fingers to form an A, you will locate the spot just above the cervix. When you stimulate the A-spot, the ejaculation is more like a river flowing and not like squirting. You have a greater volume of ejaculation coming from the A-spot, which comes from inside the yoni, whereas the G-spot ejaculation comes from urethra.

According to a paper written by Nick Fleming in 2006, called "Review of Female Ejaculation during Orgasm", Fleming writes, "The proportion of women able to ejaculate during orgasm varies greatly between studies.

Studies done by Masters and Johnson found only 4.7% of women experience the expulsion of fluid during orgasm, while some social surveys have reported up to 54% of women experiencing ejaculation (Darling et al., 1990)". It is a phenomenon recorded throughout history, still under study and has caused a lot of controversy.

Throughout history different cultures have perceived and recorded the phenomenon on female ejaculation. Despite the phenomenon being observed and recorded, the knowledge was not openly discussed due to the lack of knowledge and hence became vague. Due to recent medical curiosity and the conducted studies and the current culture being an individualistic one, many women are seeking knowledge on female ejaculation and relating it to themselves in many ways, such as holistic healing, exploring new sexual avenues, for sexual and healthy wellbeing. Deborah Sundahl says, "Women are asking for what they want and need sexually, and are likely more satisfied than ever".

She goes on further to say, "It (our sexuality) can also be used for personal transformation, physical and emotional healing, self – realization, spiritual growth, and as a way to learn about all of life and death".

As per Fleming, "Increased awareness of female ejaculation may help women and their partners feel comfortable with this phenomenon and avoid the surgery intended to eliminate it (Zaviacic and Whipple, 1993)". He goes on to say that "it is hoped that education on the subject of female ejaculation will aid women who experience this phenomenon from undergoing irreversible surgery designed to eliminate the natural sexual response".

Female ejaculation is the yoni's ultimate release of negative energies, and this is the goal that Tantric Journey wishes to accomplish. Without the female ejaculation, the yoni can never be free of negative energies. I define this "yoni crying," when the yoni is finally experiencing the long-awaited relief. The yoni is no longer blocked by negative energies, learning to let go of the traumas that were holding it back from harnessing its ultimate energies.

The key difference between an orgasm and an ejaculation within women; an orgasm is a desirable response, but only an actual ejaculation will free the yoni from the trauma that is blocking her positive energy flow. I pride myself on teaching my female clients not to be afraid of the female ejaculation. So many members of society are so eager to make women feel ashamed about this; the goal of the Tantric Journey is to help women release this shame, anger, and sadness. Only then can they experience the fulfilment and positive energy that comes from having all of your Chakras opened and your gateways unblocked from negative energies.

Can All Women Ejaculate?

With the exception of medical complication or genetic complication then it is my belief that all women have the capability to ejaculate. If a woman cannot ejaculate at present she still has the capacity to do so with the right treatment and training.

Certain studies claim that even if certain women do not ejaculate an amount of ejaculatory fluid is found in the urine after an orgasm. Therefore allowing conclusion on the fact that all women have the anatomy to ejaculate but statistics on expulsion of fluid can vary as observed by the literature provided in this report. Hence letting us arrive to a conclusion, though all women are anatomically equipped, only certain woman ejaculate. Validating the mentioned conclusion is the following text in Deborah Sundahl's book on female ejaculation:" Female ejaculation is every woman's birth right because all women are born with the anatomical ability to ejaculate".

The book by Goldstein and Davis argues that it's apt to adopt as a valid explanation giving credit to the fact anatomy can vary from woman to woman. As extracted, it quotes, "Indeed, most women do not ejaculate, and this cannot be exclusively to the inexperience or partner's incompetence. It may be due to the large differences in vaginal microanatomy among women".

As Deborah Sundahl comments, "Not all women ejaculate, nor do they need to do so in order to enjoy a life filled with sexual pleasure. Some women are natural ejaculators. Others have taught themselves to ejaculate. To make it a standard or a goal for all women would be foolish and destructive".

Yvonne K. Fulbright, author of Touch Me There! A Hands-On Guide to Your Orgasmic Hot Spots, confirms the above as she writes, "Every woman has the potential to ejaculate. Some women and their partners know it happens, others mistake it for urination, while still others remain completely uninformed about the phenomenon".

Why Some Women Don't Ejaculate

There are many reasons as to why women don't ejaculate. The following reasons are from extracted texts from various sources, which present interesting debates and explanations as to why some women don't ejaculate.

There are two main reasons attributing as main ejaculate inhibitors, (a) lack of information and knowledge is one and (b) sexual dysfunction the other.

Lack of Information and Knowledge:

Many women are ejaculate-illiterate; in other words, they simply don't know how to do it. The following are texts supporting the first main reason.

Deborah Sundahl, states, "There are important reasons why a woman doesn't ejaculate. And these primarily stem from the lack of information".

Sexual Dysfunction

Sexual dysfunction is not in direct relation to distinct anatomical flaws in women. It is with regard to other main inhibitors consisting of various elements that contribute to stalling or blocking the ejaculation. The following is an array of literature on the elements pointed out through literature extraction.

The German Ernst Gräfenberg wrote, "Although female orgasm has been discussed for many centuries or even thousands of years, the problems of female satisfaction are not yet solved......The solution of the problem would be better furthered, if the sexologists know exactly what they are talking about. The criteria for sexual satisfaction have first to be fixed..."

And he further says that "the anterior wall of the vagina along the urethra is the seat of a distinct erotogenic zone and has to be taken into account more in the treatment of female sexual deficiency".

Negative Emotions

Negative emotions in the conscious and subconscious mind play a part in acting as the blocker during an orgasm. Barry R. Komisaruk and Beverly Whipple state that "in addition to sensory factors, orgasms are often affected by cognitive, psychological, and pharmacological factors such as distraction, worry, relaxation, medication and the like".

Negative emotions can be caused due to trust related issues and physical appearance insecurity in women that they may exhibit with the partner during coitus. This can create the kind of block that makes it difficult for women to experience an orgasm.

Deborah Sundahl writes: "Traditionally, women have not been encouraged to let go and be themselves, either emotionally or physically, and the fear that they will urinate instead of ejaculate prevents many women from "letting go" when making love.

Letting go is the aspect of the female ejaculation that is most difficult for women to master. Women tend to focus so much on pleasing their men that they may forget to be selfish about their own lovemaking. Women may also be embarrassed by the process of ejaculating, which means they might feel ashamed or nervous about doing it in front of a partner.

Deep seated sexual issues can make it difficult for women to ejaculate. Awakening the G- Spot is an important step in a woman's sexual life, and it can bring up all kind of sexual issues".

These negative messages are stored physically, as memories, in the body. By understanding how this "body memory" operates, women can use a valuable physical technique that can help heal and protect them from all kinds of assaults to their sexuality, from minor to serious. Rape is a traumatic event that can shatter the ability to open and trust sexually and it can create body armouring in a woman's genitals.

Unwanted, but permitted, entry into the vagina can also cause harm, because it requires 'lies to the self' and the disassociation between the mind and body. This, too, creates emotional scars that can lodge themselves in the G–Spot, and manifest areas that are numb to touch.

Mental Social Conditioning

Cathy Winks and Anne Semans, explain the theory of mental and social conditioning in 'Sexy Mamas: Keeping Your Sex Life Alive While Raising Kids': "Your expectations and the understanding of the sexual desire are inevitably shaped by the world around you. Sure 'sexual' impulses are purely natural but the way we think and feel about them is profoundly influenced by culture".

They further write: "It is not easy to shrug off thousands of years' worth of sex – negativity. We're all raised on a steady diet of stereotypes about sex; that nice girls don't have it, that boys like sex and girls like romance, or sex is either a reproductive necessity or a shameful pleasure. As a result we live in a society of fairly ignorant and repressed sexual adults whose fascination with what have been hidden, forbidden, or denounced throughout their lives now drives a sex-obsessed economy".

"Each of us brings our entire past to every relationship. Our unique approach to sexual relationships, is shaped by a lifetime of social conditioning, religious upbringing, family values, and past sexual experiences."

This is perhaps the greatest summary that explains why some women can't ejaculate, while others can. Women are bombarded by societal pressures on a daily basis. They're constantly being told that they should act like sexual diva porn stars in bed, but they essentially shouldn't like sex.

Women are more subjected to sexual mistreatment both physical and psychological whether minor or major, of a sexual assault. Body hang-ups, societal pressures, and any negative emotion, sadness, fear etc. can contribute to a woman feeling ashamed about ejaculating, which is why it might be so difficult for her to achieve this milestone.

Through my work I have witnessed that every woman's yoni is ready to cry so that it can release the negative energies that are preventing the woman from living a satisfying and healthy life.

Orgasms aren't just limited to the yoni or the prostate; in fact, when my clients have harnessed the positive energies within their bodies, they find that their entire physical beings are capable of orgasm even at the slightest touch. This is known as an erogenous zone, as it's a sexually charged area that's capable of bringing much sexual pleasure at the slightest touch.

What Are Erogenous Zones?

Erogenous zones are specific areas in a woman's or man's body that upon touch stimulate sexual arousal. There are specific identified zones (genitals) that are always responsive in every individual on a general basis. Apart from these generally identified erogenous zones (genitals), each individual has their very own set of erogenous zones, which can be other parts of the body excluding the genitals. One's own set of erogenous zones are derived from many aspects and psychological means being one.

Erogenous zones can differ from person to person, as noted by Barry R. Komisaruk and Beverly Whipple: "For many people their erogenous zones extend beyond their genitals. The location of these zones is amazingly diverse and highly individualistic. Stimulation of an individual's 'personal erogenous zones' can greatly affect the intensity of his or her orgasms."

As per Fleming: "However, because the anterior wall of the vagina has at least three erogenous zones, Halban's fascia, the urethra and clitoral tissue, and the G-spot, stimulation of the G-spot possibly can stimulate the other erogenous areas leading to higher states of arousal and female ejaculation (Levin, 2003)".

As classified under The Arousal Sites to Trigger Orgasm (erogenous zones) by the Women's sexual function and dysfunction: study, diagnosis and treatment By Irwin Goldstein, Susan R. Davis: "The induction of female orgasm can occur from a variety of anatomic sites. These include the major ones of the clitoris (especially the glans) and the vagina (especially the anterior wall that includes Halban's fascia, the urethra and the G–Spot), but orgasm can be obtained by stimulation of the periurethral glans area (the area surrounding the urethral meatus), mons, or breast / nipples by mental or imagery fantasy, or by hypnotic suggestion. Kingsey et.al, reported that the orgasm could occur even from bizarre stimulations such as that of the teeth or blowing on the hair of the subjects. Consciousness is not a requirement".

Tantric Journey can help bring all of this into being by charging the entire body with sexual pleasure and energy; by firstly dispersing the negative emotions that are blocking this pleasure.

Raising Ecstasy Levels

A recent brain-imaging study by Swedish researchers shows that relaxation is the single most important factor in bringing a woman to orgasm.

Let's find out what stops women to relax. Women are emotionally minded while men are logically minded. Women can shut down because of negative stagnant emotions (such as shame, fear, sadness, mistrust, etc.). Also women devote a high proportion of their daily energy keeping these negative energies intact, without letting go. This makes them tired. I find as soon as they let go of such emotions they get energised and live a life with a surplus of glowing energy.

Women can easily be aroused for multi-orgasmic potential if they could get rid of the negative emotions that's blocking their creation and movement of their positive orgasmic sexual energy flow. It is not easy to get rid of them, as they are stored deeply in the body cellular memory as a result of past trauma. Whenever women are aroused they need to be present, but they lose their focus due to negative unconscious emotional waves that come and go in every moment in their lives.

These negative emotions are their protective mechanism that keep them safe, but it's the overprotection that makes them unable to even have an orgasm with their partners. In order to help her, the healer has to earn her trust with a deep connection to help her release her negative emotions by holding the space for her to release them. Once she accepts that and feels safe, she can totally relax her body and mind. At this stage, orgasm will happen without having to do much work to achieve it.

Relaxation is the most important factor in having an orgasm. There are many levels of orgasms. Many people have an orgasm at the genital level, which needs lesser relaxation. When you relax both your mind and body fully into an altered state of consciousness (otherwise known as a trance-like state), you can have a full body orgasm in the head. This is when the sexual energy is able to move from the pelvic basin to the crown via all 7 Chakras (via hormone producing glands).

Sexual energy naturally resides within us as a life-energy force that is positively charged and what prevents this energy moving into the Crown Chakra is blocked in the body as a result of stagnant emotions which creates a negatively charged energy force. These negative stagnant emotions prevent women from relaxing and enabling them to get to the orgasmic state. In Tantric Journey, I help women to relax by teaching them how to meditate with conscious breathing while I do a deeply relaxing three-hour full body massage which makes them go into a voluntary trance state, allowing them to relax their body and mind.

This Bodywork removes stagnant negative emotions embedded in the cellular memory in the pelvic area with massage techniques incorporating certain breathing patterns. Massaging the yoni gently with unconditional love will enable a woman to release such negative imprints and achieve positive mental attitude and body image.

Every woman is capable of multiple, full body orgasms with ejaculations. I have achieved this in one day for some, while others may take ten sessions or more. I am not focusing on giving an orgasm to a woman, but my focus is on removing stagnant emotions in the whole body including internal organs. Each emotional release treatment can take half a day. If I focus on her orgasm as a way of treating her, this will put further pressure on her, causing her to shut down due to negative emotions attached to the expectations.

Becoming orgasmic and / or ejaculating is only the beginning of the Journey, whereby she opens her gateway to release emotions through ejaculation. Further treatments and ejaculations will help her to unblock upper body clearing, including any issues with intimacy, love, communication, vision and spirituality, thus making her achieve full body orgasms and feel the same pleasure in her head as well as in her genitals.

If the woman has a supportive partner, this makes her process much easier, because the first problem women have is the guilt of having pleasure or betrayal after having the treatment. I find most women are extremely faithful to their partners, more so than to themselves. This is a common barrier that prevents women from coming to see me or seeking help.

Once they come to see me, it helps them to get rid of some of the guilt and shame from their cellular memory. Also they recognise that this is not a sexual treatment, but an emotional release treatment, which makes them feel sad, angry etc. when they go home. If they don't have a supportive partner, they have to suppress these negative emotions without fully experiencing them and allowing them to leave their body.

Unfortunately not many of my clients have partners who understand or trust my treatment meaning that they are unable to share with anyone if they go to see a counsellor, therapist or a psychotherapist.

Most of my clients come to see me by word of mouth but without anyone's knowledge. After a few treatments, their partners find the benefits of her renewed and heightened love, intimacy and sexuality and strengthen their relationship and the partner gets the credit for this unknown transformation.

What makes her partner behave this way is due to lack of understanding of woman's emotional blocks and not because they don't care. They also have their own insecurities thinking he will lose her if she goes for healing sessions. None of these are true and it's best for both of them to meet up with the healer and be comfortable with the environment, the healer and the treatment and ask as many questions as needed before embarking on the journey. It's best for the man to go with a Dakini (the female version of me) to help open up and to teach him how to support his partner. Once they both are healed, open and learn a new way to love, be intimate and have sex, it will transform their lives to a different level.

It is possible for a woman to self-heal without my assistance. Healing should be focused on getting rid of stagnant negative emotions from the body and allowing positive emotions to fill the vacuum.

If a woman is interested in utilising these practices to self-heal, here are my recommendations for activities and exercises she can do:

1. Any form of yoga, dance or body movements. I can highly recommend Kundalini yoga and Osho's dynamic meditation as a way of healing
2. Pelvic floor exercises incorporating breath
3. Jade egg exercises to strengthen the pelvic floor muscles
4. Meditation to still the mind
5. Breathing, Sounds (toning or Mantras) and Sound Healing to unblock emotions
6. Emotional release Deep Bodywork
7. To eat healthy (alkaline) food and to avoid an acidic environment in the body
8. To breathe fresh air
9. To be closer to nature as trees absorb negative energies from us and feed us with positive energies
10. To be around positive spiritual people and surroundings
11. Keep away from smoking, taking drugs and alcohol

12. Drink plenty of water daily, eat healthy food, exercise and sleep well

If a woman follows any of the practices that I've just listed, she may come to realize that she's capable of healing herself and unblocking most of the negative energies that are residing within her body. Of course, this takes a great amount of insight and a willingness to work through. This can't always be done by a person suffering from trauma, as they find that it's easier to go along with their lives feeling numb, rather than risk the pain, anger, and sadness that has to be released during the Tantric Journey.

Healthy Orgasm

Why are orgasms healthy?

Orgasms have been linked to the easing of arthritis, PMS and to reducing the risk of cancer. Mainstream medicine is now supporting the health giving properties of the orgasm and whilst an orgasm a day may not always keep the doctor away there are significant health and well-being benefits to be gained from experiencing orgasms.

What are the Benefits of Full Body Orgasm?

The Human Brain

- Improve body immune system and self-healing mechanism activating Stem cells (via Pineal glands)

- Release of Prolactin to enhance immune system and create a Relaxed state

- Enhance the production of Endorphins (in Pituitary Gland),making people more balanced with their Masculine-Feminine, relaxed, healthy, giving pleasure and happiness, reducing tension and stress

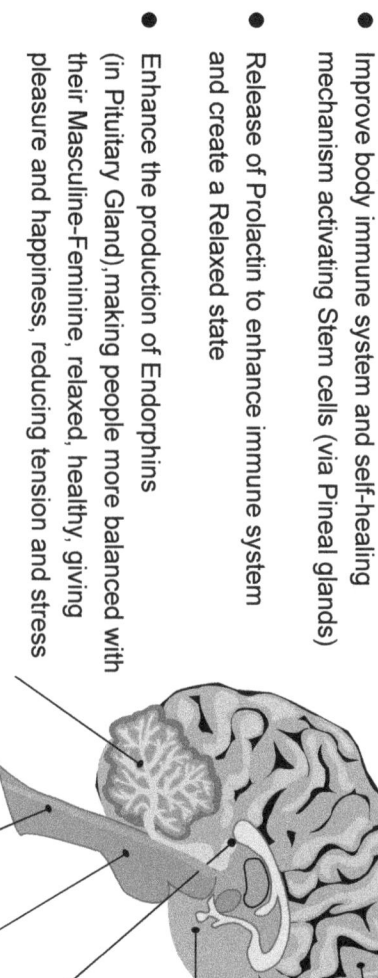

Cerebellum
(Muscle Coordination)

Spinal Cord

Brain Stem

Pineal Gland

Pituitary Gland

Cerebral Cortex
(Consciousness & memory)

When you climax there is a natural chemical rush where feel-good chemicals known as endorphins are released. These bring about a sense of euphoria, reduce stress, enhance relaxation and lead to an increased feeling of well-being. Endorphins don't just make you feel good, they have real health benefits. Endorphins are a group of substances formed within the body that naturally relieve pain. They have a similar chemical structure to morphine. In addition to their analgesic, or pain-relieving, effect, endorphins are thought to be involved in controlling the body's response to stress, regulating contractions of the intestinal wall, and determining mood. They may also regulate the release of hormones from the pituitary gland, notably growth hormone and the gonadotropin hormones.

You may wonder what all this increased blood flow and endorphin release during orgasm means for our health and well-being. Here is how it helps to revitalise our bodies and minds:

Improving Memory
and Learning

As we age, it is commonly recognised that our brain cells begin to die and it is reported that by the time we are thirty-five we are losing them at a rate of around 7,000 per day. Research has shown that stress, anxiety and depression can shrink an area of the brain known as the hippocampus which is responsible for memory and learning, but the endorphins released during orgasm stimulate the growth of new cells in the hippocampus. Scientists from Princeton University in the United States conducted an in-depth study that showed that the endorphins released during orgasm also have a positive role in protecting our brain cells against decline. "There is some evidence that older people who are sexually active are less likely to have dementia and this could be for a variety of complex reasons," says Dr Ghosh. Modern medical science has been harnessed to clinically show how the brain receives positive benefits during orgasm, "MRI scans have shown that during orgasm the neurons in the brain are more active and use more oxygen," explains Barry Komisaruk, professor of psychology at Rutgers University, "It appears that the more active the neurons, the more oxygen they withdraw from the blood — so more oxygenated blood is supplied to the region, delivering a fresh supply of nutrients."

Helps Keep you Young and Prolongs Life Expectancy

Dr David Weeks, head of old-age psychology at the Royal Edinburgh Hospital in the UK, has spent ten years studying the lifestyles of people who age prematurely, interviewing more than 3,500 people aged between 18 and 102. He discovered that couples who claimed to make love at least three times a week appeared an average ten years younger than those who had sex twice a week or less. He explains that, 'It [sex] makes us happy and produces chemicals that directly enhance the body and mind,' It's important to recognise that it's not just the amount of sex you're having that counts when it comes to adding years to your life or holding onto your youth and vitality, it's the ability to orgasm. There have been many studies conducted into the effect of orgasms leading to the discovery that orgasms can increase the body's infection-fighting cells by up to 20% and that those in fulfilled relationships live longer than singles or those in negative relationships.

Relieves Pain

Sex could be described as the 'ultimate analgesic', for it is a powerful, natural painkiller. There is strong evidence that the feel-good chemicals released by the brain during sex act as effective painkillers. During sex, blood flow increases to all parts of the body as you reach an orgasmic state, and this takes pressure away from the brain. Complete relaxation after an orgasm then reduces tension in all muscle groups, including those in the neck and back.

Enhances Mood

During an orgasm the release of a chemical called oxytocin from the pituitary gland occurs. Oxytocin flows into the body, helping to create feelings of relaxation and security. Its production continues after lovemaking, helping to create a long-term bond and aiding couples to evoke lasting memories of their sexual partner. Following sex when the blood flow has increased to the brain, a person will be more mentally alert than they were before they had sex and this in conjunction with the warm, secure emotions enhanced by the oxytocin leads to mood enhancement.

Reduces PMS

Orgasm has been shown to help regulate oestrogen levels in women and a few studies have shown it is important in controlling the menstrual cycle and may even reduce PMS (premenstrual syndrome).

Aids Natural Sleep Patterns

One of the chemicals released during orgasm is prolactin, which is linked to the feeling of sexual satisfaction but also leads to aiding sleep. This combined with all the relaxation benefits that an orgasm provides has led to the orgasm being dubbed a natural cure for insomnia.

As all of this research suggests, a healthy orgasm is one of the best ways for women to feel better about themselves and it has many health and well-being benefits. Orgasmic energy is a positively charged energy force. When it travels through the body and meets any negatively charged cells, it transforms into a positive charged cell making our body more positive, loving and healthy.

During a full body orgasm the body will experience spasm. This is a way of dispersing stuck negative energy from the body and making way for the positive orgasmic energy to move towards the Crown Chakra and out of body.

A full body orgasm is a revitalising experience because when it reaches the brain and stimulates the pineal gland, it activates stem cells in the body to start repairing and healing the body where needed. Full body orgasm is our natural body healing mechanism.

Deeply Fulfilling Relationships

Tantric Journey can help produce a deeply fulfilling and loving relationship. My female clients are given the knowledge and empowerment they need to approach lovemaking in a healthier and happier manner. After the 'yoni cries', these women are suddenly free from the negative experiences and energies that were causing them to be so sad and angry all the time.

Suddenly, these women are happier mothers, happier wives, happier friends, and happier co-workers. They're no longer being weighed down by the negative experiences they've had in their lives before. They're suddenly opening up to new experiences, and engaging in a journey with their partner that's full of tenderness and intimacy. They're like a flower blossoming, and their lover is like the bee that's coming to drink the pollen. It's a beautiful and satisfying part of doing what I do, because I'm helping these people have the kind of healthy, intimate, and loving relationships that they've always wanted, but didn't know how to get.

That's why I often invite clients' husbands to come into a session to see what I do. I find that even though I don't perform the massages on men, they find that their partners are so transformed by the healing experiences of the massage that they're instantly aware of why the Tantric Journey is so critical. It's just another way these men become truly loving and supporting partners, thus leading to a fulfilling relationship.

Surviving a Healing Crisis

A healing crisis can be an unpleasant and often painful experience. It is a common occurrence following healing or Bodywork and I consider a healing crisis the growing pains of the emotional detox work I perform.

In Eastern medicine and holistic approaches to healing, a "healing crisis", (or Herxheimer Reaction), is marked as a sign that the modality being used is having a balancing effect. When the body starts to detox and heal itself, it sometimes isn't able to release toxins fast enough and various symptoms can appear. Whilst these symptoms will pass they can at times feel intense.

In Western medicine symptoms of any kind are usually viewed as bad and the focus is to get rid of the symptom. Many of us have become detached from the concept that our body has the ability to heal itself, and instead look to cure symptoms with medication. Bodywork of any sort, energy work, physical detox, emotional detox and improvements in nutrition can all cause reactions, which are in fact signs of improvement and is actually your body's way of processing the treatment.

Experiencing a healing crisis following a Tantric Journey treatment is a completely normal response that many of my clients go through; the effects of my treatment could be likened to a traumatic event such as the sudden death of a loved one. The effect of my treatment is so powerful that my clients can feel emotions stronger than they have ever experienced before. They might sob uncontrollably every minute of the day – with an intensity never felt before. They may feel physical pain from the emotion. They may feel they are over the edge of sanity and are totally out of control. Whilst others describe having a 'break down'. In reality what is really happening is a 'break through' as they smash through a layer of negative emotional baggage and begin to clear stagnant emotions through emotional detox.

While it may hurt and it may be confusing, it can also feel quite energising to let go of the emotions and allow your sadness to drain away in your tears. All the emotions that have been bottled up inside are suddenly flushed outward – finally the beginning of freedom is in progress.

It is frightening to let go and feel out of control. The fact that one treatment has pushed you into a healing crisis can make you wary of the treatment and blame the therapist. Suddenly you are unsure of everything. You are constantly reminded of how important it is to stay in control at all times, yet you also know that it feels so good to let go. You may experience a sense of chaotic disharmony for a while before you can process this new experience.

Each treatment session unravels the layers of physical and emotional holding within the body. This is the equivalent of peeling away the many layers of an onion. As the outer layers unfold the next layer presents itself to us as an untold story, where new emotions are stored and new information is revealed. In the short term it is always easier not to face up to our problems, but in the long term emotional blockages will lead to disease.

When going through a healing crisis you may experience physical symptoms. Your shoulders may ache, you may develop crippling back pain or joint discomfort. You could develop cold or flu symptoms and you may feel weak as shame and guilt overtake you. This is all part of the healing process and you may feel worse before you feel better as your whole body readjusts itself to the changes that the healing is initiating.

In order to gain a real understanding of the healing crisis, it is important to understand the theory of the wounding crisis and how this affects our body. A wounding experience is a physical or emotional memory that is stored within the cellular memory of the body. A wounding crisis can occur as a result of a major trauma or over time accumulating like water from a dripping tap. The three primary forces that help to create a wounding crisis are stress, repression, and physical trauma.

The Three Primary Forces

Stress

Stress can become a force in our lives when we do not feel safe. Periods of unrest can allow stress to hijack our minds and body. Stress is primarily an emotional experience. Through fear our body reacts into the Fight or Flight Response discussed earlier in this book. This primitive mechanism is purely designed to keep us alive. Our primary instinct is to survive. When we go into a stressed state our muscles hold on to it in a pre-set pattern, perhaps around the jaw, eyes, in the shoulders or in the back of the neck. Over time and with repeated activation these same muscles tend to harden and bond together, causing physical pain. In a way, the layers of our tissues, just like the layers of an onion, become cemented together because we cannot expel the emotion. It is the molecules of emotions that make our muscles contract hoping to protect ourselves from danger.

Repression

Repression is another emotion that exists in the wounding crisis. Repression occurs when we use our own muscular system to hold back the energy of our emotions without dispersing at the time of occurrence. Over time repetitive behaviour and the repression of emotion leads to the layers of muscles hardening and bonding together. When clients feel deep sadness after Bodywork it is because the treatment is rupturing years of repression stored within the cellular memory of their muscles.

Physical Trauma

Physical trauma is the third primary force involved in a wounding crisis. This can be as the result of accidents, physical abuse, falls, car accidents or any other physical trauma. The energy of impact for example in domestic violence is unable to dissipate and will be stored within the body. There is nothing to absorb the trauma, nowhere for it to go, so the only place the energy can go is into your own body.

It is not just a large physical trauma such as a blow to the head that is stored; smaller, repetitive traumas can accumulate over time. Repetitive physical trauma will build up like a layer of lime scale with the energy of every single blow that your body receives being lodged within your cellular memory.

The strain of stress, repression and physical trauma will over time result in a wounding crisis. Under our current belief system we tend to hold on tightly when we are injured or feel the effects of stress. We clench and hold on firmly to the negative emotions and trauma, we keep our muscles tight and the area immobilized, thus locking the trauma into our body.

With a lockdown at the site of trauma eventually the brain stops sending nerve impulses to this area. The areas that we hold onto tightly begin to lose sensation and become numb. I have treated many women who have had no feeling in their yoni through holding on tightly to the traumas of sexual abuse or negative relationships or traumatic childbirth. In the area of the body where we have almost clenched so hard that it is blocked, we begin to lose our ability to feel the memory stored in the region because we have desensitized the area. This is a clever coping mechanism in many respects, but it is not a long term solution because we do not feel better because we no longer feel pain. All it means is that we have rendered an area redundant and barren; we have stopped the energy flow and the area has lost sensation. Over time the layers of muscles and soft tissue remain motionless and immobilized and a layer of "armour" forms. The wound is still there and whilst we try to ignore the pain and cover it up with layers of de-sensitisation and armouring, we are still holding on to the wounding experiences.

In short if trauma is not released as soon as possible after it has occurred, then it will be stored in the body and, as you carry the emotional weight of armouring, it will manifest in things such as excess weight, hardened muscles, hardened soft tissue, trust issues, depression and other behavioural or physical ailments.

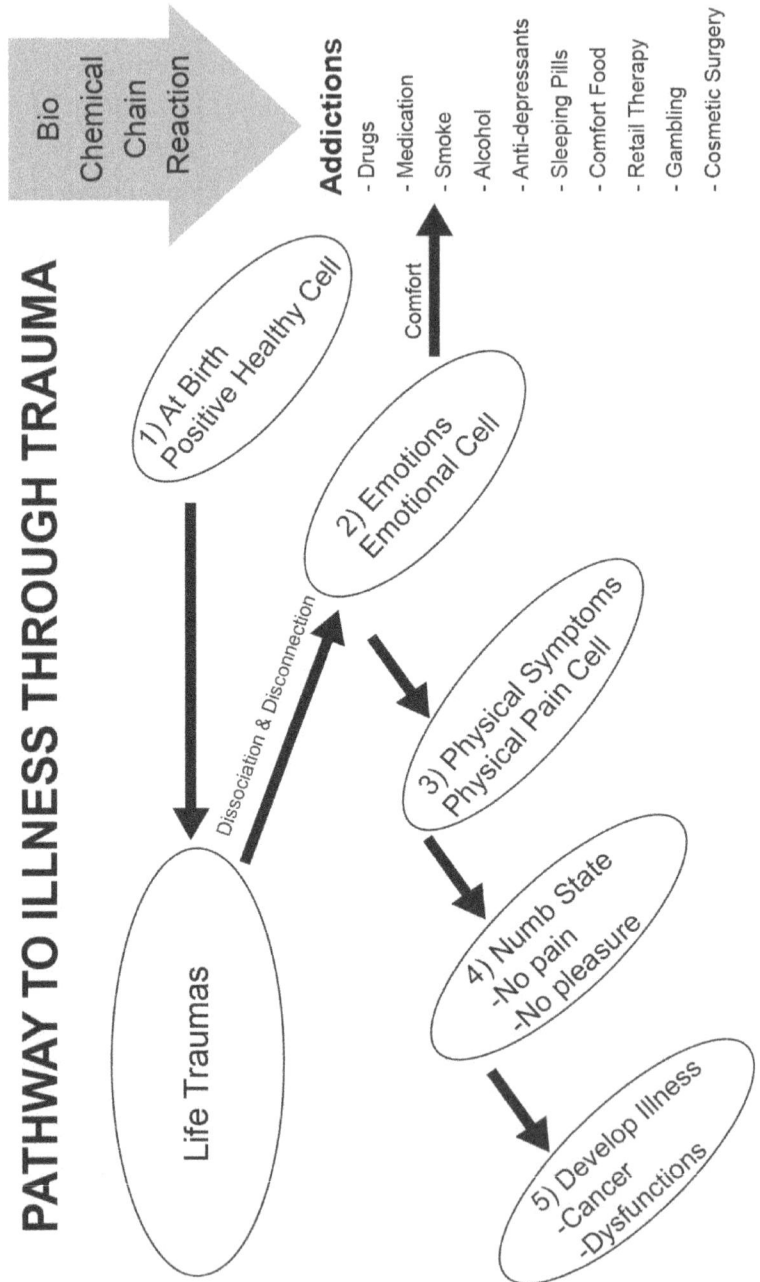

PATHWAY TO ILLNESS THROUGH TRAUMA

Bio Chemical Chain Reaction

1) At Birth Positive Healthy Cell

Life Traumas

Dissociation & Disconnection

2) Emotions Emotional Cell

Comfort

Addictions
- Drugs
- Medication
- Smoke
- Alcohol
- Anti-depressants
- Sleeping Pills
- Comfort Food
- Retail Therapy
- Gambling
- Cosmetic Surgery

3) Physical Symptoms Physical Pain Cell

4) Numb State
  -No pain
  -No pleasure

5) Develop Illness
  -Cancer
  -Dysfunctions

Unpeeling the Body's Onion

The work I do peels away the layers of trapped negative emotion that have been frozen in time and this can prompt the healing crisis to occur. When we begin to strip away layers of armour through Bodywork, it can be as significant and painful as the original trauma because the first stage of a healing crisis is to come out of numbness and bring back sensation and emotion to the body. If you have been numb for years, it can be frightening when the sensations arise. Coming out of numbness into sensation is the first step in healing, but it can be a daunting process.

Imagine all the cells in your body are represented by a box filled with emotions. During a Tantric Journey session, the lid on this box gets opened allowing the trapped negative emotions to escape. This release may take place during the session and after the session; indeed it is usual for this to continue for up to three days after treatment. During this period the lid of the box is still open and it slowly shuts down to its original positon. Three days after treatment you will be less negative and feel more positive and alive. The healing recovery process will depend on the amount of blocks one has and the intensity of the treatment. Some clients have taken over 2-3 weeks to recover and there is no way of telling how long recovery will take. Release comes in many forms and these are displayed below:

How You May Feel After a Session

- Feel Sad (Crying for days)
- Feel Frustrated
- Feel Angry and Rage
- Feel Shame
- Feel Mistrust
- Feel Guilty
- Feel Dirty and Disgust
- Feel Doubt
- Feel Abused

- Headaches
- Spots appear on the face
- Spots appear on the body
- An Illness
- Tummy Aches
- Severe body aches
- See bad dreams
- Feel Depressed
- Body Shaking

It is important to acknowledge the release and fully feel all the emotions, as and when they come as waves in the sea. Breathe into them and let go. Be in a positive and supporting environment, drink lots of water, keep a hot water bottle, if the yoni or tummy aches, eat and drink non-toxic food between the sessions. Keep away from smoking, alcohol, drugs, pain killers etc. as they suppress and numb the evoked emotions and put it back into the body.

Emotional Release

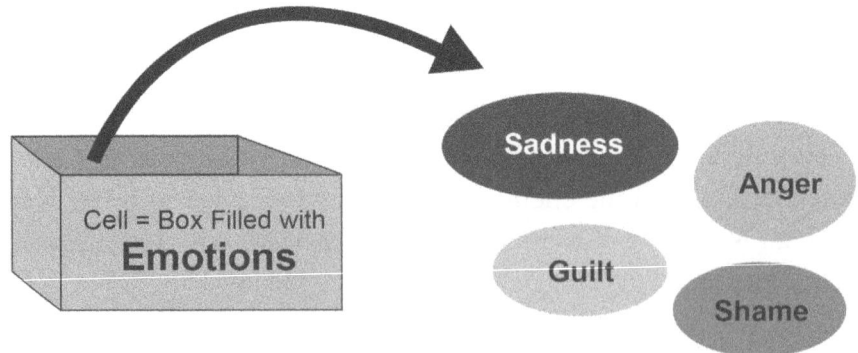

Unfortunately, most mainstream medical professionals and professional therapists are not trained in how to understand the healing crisis. It is a very important part of the healing process, but is often overlooked or misunderstood with a healing crisis being labelled as a symptom of a "breakdown or insane", or of abuse or disease. When people turn to medical professionals for help with their healing crisis, they are often medicated in order to suppress the symptoms. Some individuals going through a healing crisis might be tempted to turn to alcohol, tobacco or drugs to supress their emotions. Whilst all of these may help to lessen the intensity of the experience, it will only supress the emotions and stop the healing process.

Many people, who have experienced traumatic events in their life, live their life without feeling and find solace in their numbness. Then when physical and emotional symptoms manifest, they seek help but the road to recovery can be unpleasant and very painful in the beginning.

The symptoms of a healing crisis can include pain, pressure, and lack of coordination. Whilst other symptoms include frequent urination, heavy sweating, depression, explosive anger, extreme sadness and even vomiting or diarrhoea. The body during these times tends to enter into a state of chaos with extreme tiredness and fever symptoms being common.

A healing crisis is a profound experience where the body is able to expel stored emotions and begin to regain equilibrium. Donald Epstein writes in Healing Myths Healing Magic, "Once again, disease is not a mistake of a stupid body; it is the body's attempt to reorganise its energy systems to allow for a greater exchange of information and energy and thus a greater expression of consciousness."

The healing crisis should not be repressed, but embraced as our body is attempting to come back to balance and harmony. The healing crisis is not creating new problems for the body but releasing the issues that are lying dormant deep below the surface. As the body attempts to unblock that which is blocked and return us back to our natural flow we can often feel at our lowest ebb, but it will pass and when it has we will feel restored and nurtured.

Donald Epstein writes in Healing Myths Healing Magic, "Healing occurs the instant a physical or mechanical obstruction is removed, or the instant we express our inner wisdom. Healing occurs the instant that parts of our body begin to share their stories with one another. Healing occurs the moment we liberate blocked energy that is stored in different areas of our body, or when our breath becomes more easy and natural."

When experiencing a healing crisis after treatment we should never attempt to block it, but trust in the experience and go with the healing flow. There are no rules about the symptoms that will be experienced or the time that it will take. Emma Bragdon writes on the question of how long it will take in 'The Call of Spiritual Emergency,' "There is no answer to this. It depends on what kind of patterns of spiritual emergence people are experiencing. If the experience is physically very intense, it will end when the body gets tired of the intensity. Likewise, if it is very emotional, the crisis will let up when the body tires of catharsis. All life pulsates, expands and contracts. A contraction cycle will inevitably follow an expansion. An expansion will inevitably follow a contraction."

How to Handle a Healing Crisis?

1. Seek a safe and supportive environment. Find support with loved ones or family and avoid negative individuals.
2. Ask for help from positive supportive people who understand the healing process. It is almost impossible to take care of yourself in the same manner when experiencing a healing crisis.
3. Keep a journal. Sometimes writing down your thoughts and feelings is a good way of processing.
4. Surrender to the experience. Do not fight the process or try to rationalise it. Just go with it and allow yourself time and space to process your healing.
5. Avoid toxins and stimulants. Try not to use food or other addictions to suppress these new feelings and sensations. Try to eat a natural, vegetarian diet and drink plenty of water.
6. Get out into nature. Walking and enjoying the peace and healing harmony of nature can be helpful when processing and feeling the need for sanctuary.
7. Take time to nurture yourself. Meditation and relaxation practices are deeply helpful.
8. Avoid falling into depression. Depression takes hold when the energy of emotion does not flow out of us. Walking, tai chi, gentle swimming and yoga can be very helpful, but avoid strenuous exercise.
9. Above all be kind to yourself and focus on positive meditations.

What Tantric Journey Offers

The Deep Bodywork that l carry out in a Tantric Journey healing session will help to dissolve negative thoughts, feelings, emotions, actions, issues and blocks and will create sufficient positive energies that will spread throughout your body to heal every cell.

This treatment gives the client ultimate control of the pace and focus of the healing. Tantric Journey teaches the body and mind to self-heal, self-develop and to master the skills of achieving a full body, extended Multi Orgasmic Response (MORE), instead of a localized genital release, putting the woman in charge of her own sexuality, instead of depending on a man, woman or even a vibrator for that release.

You can read more about my work as a therapist on my website: http://www.tantricjourney.com

Courses and Training Workshops

In addition to private sessions available in London, UK, Tantric Journey is shared through a program of talks, workshops and retreats held globally.

It begins with 'The Tantric Journey weekend Workshop', a beginner's course where you get to roll up your sleeves and experience the easy-to-master yet extremely potent healing and transformational foundational tools. You then move on to the more advanced events, which deepen your experience and challenge the boundaries of what we thought we knew to be true and to recognise the true potential and boundless possibilities available to each of us in true freedom.

For those of you willing to dive in even deeper, the Certified Tantric Journey Educator Program will strip away the illusions upon which your life has been based, uncovering blocks and penetrating the lies, leaving you soaring as an expression of freedom, enabling you to be certified as a Tantric Journey Educator and facilitate healing for others.

Each of my comprehensive events is a once in a lifetime experience and offers you the most up-to-date, in depth and transformational healing available anywhere -- profoundly healing seminars and retreats where you clear issues that have held you back from allowing your full potential to flourish.

These events provide cutting edge skills and liberating process work that will powerfully and positively transform every area of your life. They offer the ability to free yourself from life-long issues leaving you soaring and living a life in joy, wholeness and peace.

This program allows you to be a beacon of healing and transformational possibility, a catalyst for the change our world needs NOW – because ultimately,

As Gandhi once said,

> *"YOU are the change you wish to see in the world" - Gandhi*

For classes - Workshops - Private Sessions
www.tantricjourney.com

About the Author

Mal is a British Pioneer in the Area of Emotional Release through Bodywork, who has studied in various accredited institutes under pioneers and experts earning him the accolade of being the first Certified Tantra Educator in the UK (from Source School of Tantra).

Mal has worked in the field of Human Sexuality and Emotional Detox since 1994, both in learning and treating over 3000 clients from all walks of life. Mal was invited to The Connection Conference in the Netherlands, (Rotterdam) at the Spiritual Centre Djoj, to present, 'Secrets of Female Sexuality' in December 2011 and he is invited to give talks and workshops in Tantra Festivals all over the world.

His work was embraced and recognised as hugely valuable in treating sexual dysfunction in women. Through his unique work, Mal treats sexual dysfunctions instigated by deeply rooted problems. Mal has helped to release many women from their negative emotional restraints and open a new gateway of self-actualisation.

His research, dedication and skill in sexual healing and relationship therapy has led him to treating thousands of women from around the world. Mal also travels internationally sharing and teaching, his knowledge on Tantra through presentations and master classes. The majority of his new clients are gained through existing client recommendation, which bears testimony to the effectiveness of his treatments.

Having studied at the International Centre for Release and Integration in Mill Valley, California, studying under late Dr Jack Painter, the pioneer of Postural Integration and Deep Bodywork in the USA, Mal has gained valuable knowledge and understanding.

He also studied at Source School of Tantra in Maui, Hawaii under Charles and Caroline Muir for two years, giving him his CTE certificate and becoming the first Advance Certified Tantra Educator in the UK.

Mal has also studied with Margo Anand, Bradon Bays and Grand Master Mantak Chia.

Answering your Questions: An Interview with Mal

Q. What would you say to anyone who feels uncomfortable with the theories, ideas or techniques that they have read about in this book?

A. I recognise the discomfort some of you may feel after reading this book. In many ways, we are all living a great lie. My intention in writing this is an invitation to allow you to begin to live in your truth, for then you may value what I say herein. You will then begin to listen, appreciate, understand and implement to improve the quality of your life, because I believe that we only have one life which is very short and it's only a blink away, in terms of the universal clock.

Q. When healing women what results have you witnessed?

A. When treating women I have witnessed personal transformation and empowerment. I have seen my clients taken to new levels of life with increased vitality. They flourish and create the life they want to live and I am privileged to be part of their development.

Q. What does Tantric Journey School offer?

A. Tantric Journey School offers workshops, talks and private coaching sessions for individuals and couples. Tantric Journey is a therapy that includes a potent mix of Tantra, Tao, breath work, sound, movement, energy work, Deep Bodywork and other therapies to open and balance as well as attune and develop. The school also offers a 10 day certified Tantric Journey Educator Program.

Q. What got you interested in Tantra?

A. For me it was a path I recognised as being one that would support me to fulfilling my full potential. I am a natural born healer and my training has awakened my natural healing skills and has given me knowledge and consciousness that has flowed throughout all areas of my life. Over the past twenty years Spirituality and Tantra has created a deep transformation in me and continues to support my unfolding and continual development. Tantra is not something you learn about or follow, it is a way of life and it has enriched my existence through a deeper understanding of life. I am so fortunate to be sharing this path of Tantra, my knowledge and my deep commitment to it through sessions and teaching to support others on their journey of growth.

Q. What are the benefits of Tantra?

A. Tantra can benefit every area of your life. Whether you find yourself longing for fulfilment in love, sexuality, intimacy, confidence, career, creativity, release, freedom, self-realisation, empowerment, health, wealth, happiness or relationship. Whatever it is you are seeking in life, Tantra can support you to experience it. I'm not suggesting that Tantra is some sort of miracle key that can unlock your deepest desires in an instant, but with time, training and healing you will open and grow and you will watch yourself evolve and develop a deeper connection with yourself, others and life.

Q. Do you think Tantra is misunderstood in Western Society?

A. Work in the Tantric field is largely misunderstood and for many, the misunderstanding is that sexual arousal and fantastic sex are the main focus of Tantra. This misconception stems from the fact that Tantra accepts sexual energy and harnesses it as a route to altered state of consciousness. This has been largely misinterpreted in the West as meaning Tantra merely focuses on achieving sexual ecstasy. It is this altered state of consciousness that helps my clients to be connected from disassociated past trauma and help let go of the negative stagnate emotions attached to the trauma. This is the trauma release work that I do which is sadly misunderstood. Tantra has subsequently gained a reputation of being outside the pale of respectability and in the minds of many, it brands female Tantric Healers as sex workers and male Tantric healers as sexual predators. The fact that Tantra treats sexual energy as an ally, rather than something to be suppressed or hushed up makes many people feel uncomfortable with the concept of the therapy. This stems from lack of understanding. Tantric work does not deny sexual energy, it embraces sexual energy, but that does not mean unenlightened media defined sex.

In the work I do, sexual energy is used as ignition for firing the Kundalini energy, the body's biological energy system, merging it with universal energy. Indeed the work I do can help a person enjoy their sex life to its fullest potential, but it is far wider reaching than that. It can help to break down barriers of guilt or fear, and remove self-imposed or limiting cultural and social boundaries and to empower women.

This is nothing to do with Sting and all night sex sessions; this is about personal development and spiritual growth. The word Tantra is a Sanskrit word which means, to weave, to transform through methods, and to transform poison into nectar. This description of Tantra offers a far better insight into the true transformational nature of the discipline. My work is all about helping people to gain release from negative trauma and transform their life, emerging like a butterfly from a chrysalis.

Q. Are there risks to the practitioner in your line of work.

A. Yes, performing Bodywork such as mine can be a risky business. During my time as a practitioner I have learned many things about safe working practices for the therapist, but I also I learned that it's not the therapist who heals the client during Deep Bodywork, but it's the client who heals herself, in the presence of a trusting therapist. The therapist only acts as a catalyst to help the client to access past trauma and stagnant negative imprints. The purpose of the treatment is to help the client to access old trauma, meeting her inner child and stagnant emotions by working on trigger points where the trauma is stored. Once the emotions are fully felt in the client's body, it's a certain deep breathing technique that enables her to release and unblock the stagnant negative emotions. She may feel fear, sadness, anger etc. during the treatment as a result of Deep Bodywork. When treatments go wrong, it is due to lack of understanding of our own bodies and emotions and also trauma transference and projections.

I now recognise that traumatised clients are more vulnerable to experiencing 'emotional pain' during Bodywork and also that there is a risk of transference, where the client can come to blame the therapist for the negative feelings they harbour.

Performing a massage on someone who is suffering emotional trauma can be likened to cracking an egg shell. Touching the body is incredibly painful and 'damaging' as the outer body is not strong enough to hold on to emotions in response to Deep Bodywork. When a male therapist like myself is performing deep, healing Bodywork, it is possible for women to become confused about the intentions of that therapist and the purpose of the work and it may awaken feelings of past abuse. Since 2005 I have studied the effects of trauma transference and have changed my working practices, I now only offer Tantric Journey treatments and no longer practice massage as a stand-alone treatment in beauty salons.

People think of massage therapy as a "safe" therapy, and for majority of the time it is. Therapists often spend a long time ensuring that their clients are in a safe and secure environment, but commonly fail to ensure their own safety as a therapist. Things can go wrong, with massage techniques being misinterpreted, clients that are suffering from emotional and psychological difficulties being the most susceptible to feelings of vulnerability. The therapist works with the client's comfort in mind. The idea is to access the muscles efficiently, not to take voyeuristic advantage of your nakedness. It's not that a massage therapist doesn't care in a callous way, it's that they view your body in a professional, matter of fact way. They are treating you; they are working on your muscles as they have worked on many bodies before and their aim is to treat you effectively.

The fact is that an ethical and responsible healer, properly trained, is just not interested in seeing your nudity. When they are looking, it's from a clinical perspective. The skin is an organ like all the others, and offers a great deal of information on what's going on inside you from an evaluative perspective.

Some of the feelings that clients may experience following Bodywork are listed on page212 and they may feel worse than before the treatment. If a client is not fully aware of the healing crises, she may doubt the treatment or blame the therapist, (especially if the therapist is a man) for the way she feels. This is one of the biggest dangers of this type of Bodywork when a man is working on female clients.

There is another danger to this work and this is called Empathy. A client may go home and release emotions for a few days, her energy changes during the healing process and friends and relatives surrounding her will notice the change and will get concerned. If these people also carry negative emotions with them, clients' emotional release can trigger their emotions and this is even more dangerous than what the client feels as they judge and make so many negative assumptions towards the therapist and the treatment based on their life experiences. In this situation when the therapist has never met them or treated them, he is unable to help them or to defend his work. This happens with Empathy, where the client's negative emotions are transferred to the people around her who are also negative. The best way to deal with this situation is for them to see the therapist himself and to have a consultation and for an explanation.

On the other hand if the client is surrounded by supportive, positive, spiritual people, this could help her to process much faster without having to explain to anyone how she feels. Once she completes her emotional process cycle, she is able to transfer her positive energy to heal and help other negative people around her.

As a practitioner I have developed a few safety methods as follows:

1. Always, I get the client to read my Tantric Journey Brochure, Treatment card and the website, that explain all the features and benefits of the treatment
2. I then speak to them via Skype, over the phone or at our first meeting to explain the features and benefits of the treatment
3. I get all my clients to sign a consent form and also offer a female chaperone if they wish to have one during the treatment
4. During the initial consultation I establish

    a. What the client wants to achieve from Tantric Journey
    b. What her boundaries are
    c. What her fears are

5. Then I work around her needs to help her achieve what she wants

6. It's always good to follow the treatment plan below but it may change from client to client. The purpose of treating this way is to release emotions in small doses, otherwise the client will be too overwhelmed and the release will be too traumatic

   a. Start with talking therapy
   b. Follow it with Yoga, Body movements and Pelvic floor exercises, Chanting, Breath work
   c. Offer a fully clothes on massage
   d. Offer a full body oil massage excluding yoni massage
   e. Offer a full body massage including yoni healing through female ejaculation
   f. Explore the 5 sensors of intimacy as a giver and as a receiver. Conscious touch, smell, hearing and talking (affirmations), eye gazing and tasting the body
   g. Explore unconditional love and modalities of kissing
   h. Giving a voice to Yoni, to open Throat Chakra

7. It is a good practice to text or e-mail the client, after the session to find out how she feels, and if I can help her in any way with her emotional release. This is very important especially during the first few sessions where the emotional release is at its highest level, especially after a yoni massage.

Q. Does it anger you that people may misconceive you and your work?

A. There will always be people who will question the validity of my work, because it challenges everything they have ever known to be true. It never angers me because everyone is entitled to make up their own minds. My work is very unique and challenges previous thoughts and treatment methods practiced in the West, so of course I expect to come under scrutiny and suspicion. My only hope is to educate people to a greater understanding of my work and its benefits.

Q. What advice would you give to any therapist starting out in the field of tantric Bodywork?

A. There have been many other cases where masseurs have been accused of preying on women during massage. For example Daniel Pytlarz recently became a high profile case in London, where eighteen women accused him of 'bad touching'. He was acquitted. I on the other hand had two complaints and was found guilty. All I can say is that massage and Bodywork is quite unlike any other treatment. It involves a level of intimacy that can easily be misinterpreted and the therapist needs to take precautions. He or she must ensure that consent forms are signed for each treatment and be aware that they must check throughout the treatment if the client is still ok, as consent can be withdrawn at any stage during the treatment.

The therapist needs to get written, verbal and energetic consent throughout the treatment as women's emotions are flowing like waves in the sea. One must listen to her body language, breathing, sounds and eye movements as ways of non-verbal communications.

When the client is triggered with a past trauma, she goes into a freeze state, making her unable to speak or even open her eyes. I have developed an NLP technique to communicate with the client in these situations. I ask her to guide me with a hand signal during the massage. If she feels uncomfortable or overwhelmed with the massage, when she does not know how to communicate verbally she will close her fist. Then I will back off from the area I was massaging or reduce the intensity.

Similarly if she wants tell me that she is having so much pleasure with what I am doing and she does not know how to tell me not to stop it. In this situation I ask her to open her hand wide open to signal me with this request and I will then work on that area longer without making any changes. I find this is a great way to ride the emotional wave with the client without them complaining about my work as she will have the control in her own hands. This also helps them to let go as they feel they are in control.

It is a rewarding line of work, but it is also a line of work that carries many risks, but these risks can be managed. You must read the chapter entitled, Healing Crisis to fully understand why this occurs in Bodywork.

Q. why is the Yoni referred to as 'she' in the book, as if it has an identity?

A. The yoni is worshipped as the sacred symbol of the Divine Feminine, referred to as the Devi, the Great Goddess, the source of life, the Universal Womb. It is the gateway to feminine sacredness and where we find universal creative energy.

Q. Is yoni massage just about bringing a woman to orgasm?

A. No. It's about helping a woman to evoke and release her trapped negative emotions and trauma from the body cellular memory, that is blocking the orgasms. Orgasms are only sign posts of Tantric Journey.

If you focus on giving an orgasm to a woman it moves away from the woman like a mirage, while the Tantric Journey makes the mirage come closer to the woman effortlessly.

Q. In your workshops what can people expect?

A. The workshops are mainly held at my beautiful Tantra Temple, although I do travel around the UK / Europe and the rest of the world to teach. Each workshop is tailored for the students attending, for example, I run beginner's classes, advanced teacher training and couple workshops. The courses will include breath work, body movement, energy work, healing, massage and the use of all senses, male female polarity work, single, partner and group Tantra practices, exploration of sexual energy and love and intimacy, meditation, sound therapy, sharing, teaching, practical work and training. The wide variety of approaches makes the work both vivid and profound.

There is no nudity in the workshops other than the model I use to show the demonstrations. All practical work that is carried out is done in your own privacy and all participants are taught to respect each other's boundaries with all sharing kept confidential.

Attendees are expected to stay away from toxic foods, drinks and toxic substances during the workshops and to abstain from sex to help build up the energy.

These classes will illuminate inward connection and also enhance deep connection with others.

Q. Do I have to bring a partner with me to experience Tantric Journey?

A. Some come alone, some with a partner; but all as individuals seeking to discover, experience and grow.

Q. How do I decide which teacher or healer is right for me?

A. There are many approaches to Tantra and there are many different practitioners across the globe. It can be confusing as to what Tantra is and what different schools, healers and teachers are offering. I have in depth articles on my website that may help people get an idea of Tantric Journey and my approach to Tantra. www.tantricjourney. co.uk

Further Reading

Below is a list of books I highly recommend:

Acupressure for Lovers: Secrets of Touch for Increasing Intimacy by Michael Reed Gach

Better Health through Natural Healing: Successful Remedies for Over 100 Common Ailments by Ross Trattler

Beyond Orgasm by Marty Klein

Cell Talk: Talking to your Cell(f) by John E. Upledger

Chi Nei Tsang: Chi Massage for the Vital Organ by Mantak Chia

Chi Nei Tsang II: Internal Organs Chi Massage, Chasing the Wind by Mantak Chia

Compersion: Meditation on Using Jealousy As A Path To Unconditional Love by Dr. Deborah Taj Anapol

Coping with Anxiety and Depression by Shirley Trickett

Deep Bodywork and Personal Development: Harmonizing Our Bodies, Emotions and Thoughts by Dr. Jack W. Painter

Emotional Anatomy by Stanley Keleman

Energy Medicine: The Scientific Basis by James L. Oschman

Erotic Massage: The Tantric Touch of Life by Kenneth Ray Stubbs & Louise-Andree Saulnier; Illustrated by Kyle Spencer

Female Ejaculation & the G-Spot by Deborah Sundahl

Freeing the Female Orgasm: Awakening the Goddess by Charles & Caroline Muir

Healing Love through the Tao: Cultivating Female Sexual Energy by Mantak Chia & Maneewan Chia

How to Be a Great Lover by Lou Paget

How to Give Her Absolute Pleasure: Totally Explicit Techniques Every Woman Wants Her Man To Know by Lou Paget

Karsai Nei Tsang: Therapeutic Massage for the Sexual Organs by Mantak Chia

Law of Attraction: Getting More of What You Want and Less of What You Don't by Michael Losier

Liberated Orgasm: The Orgasmic Revolution by Herbert A. Otto

Molecules of Emotion by Dr. Candace B. Pert

Orgasm: Over 100 Truly Explosive Tips by Lisa Sussman

Quantum Healing: Exploring the Frontiers of Mind/Body/Medicine by Deepak Chopra

Secret Sexual Positions: Ancient Techniques for Modern Lovers by Kenneth Ray Stubbs; Illustrated by Kyle Spencer

Sexual Ecstasy: The Art of Orgasm by Margot Anand

Sexual Energy Ecstasy: A Practical Guide to Lovemaking Secrets of East and West by David & Ellen Ramsdale

Sexual Healing: A Self-Help Program to Enhance Your Sensuality and Overcome Common Sexual Problems by Barbara Keesling

Sexual Healing Through Yin & Yang: Using Sexual Energy for Health, Longevity, and Enjoyment by Zaihong Shen

Sexual Health and Erotic Freedom by Barnaby B. Barratt

Sexual Reflexology: Activating the Taoist Points of Love by Mantak Chia & William U. Wei

Sexual Secrets: The Alchemy of Ecstasy by Nik Douglas & Penny Slinger

Spiritual Healing: A Beginners Guide by Kristyna Arcarti

Tantra & the Tao: The Secrets of Sexual Ecstasy by Gilly Smith

Tantra: The Art of Conscious Loving by Charles and Caroline Muir

Tantric Awakening: A Woman's Initiation into the Path of Ecstasy by Valerie Brooks

Taoist Secrets of Love: Cultivating Male Sexual Energy by Mantak Chia, Michael Winn

The 13 Secrets by Robert Denryck

The Art of Erotic Massage by Dr Andrew Yorke

The Art of Everyday Ecstasy: The Seven Tantric Keys for Bringing Passion, Spirit and Joy into Every Part of Your Life by Magot Anand

The Art of Sexual Ecstasy: The path of Sacred Sexuality for Western Lovers by Margo Anand

The Art of Sexual Magic: How to Use Sexual Energy to Transform Your Life by Margo Anand

The Complete Idiot's Guide to Tantric Sex by Dr. Judy Kuriansky

The Function of the Orgasm by Dr. Wilhelm Reich, translated by Vincent R. Carfagno

The Journey: An extraordinary Guide for Healing Your Life and Setting Yourself Free by Brandon Bays

The Multi-Orgasmic Couple by Mantak Chia & Maneewan Chia, Douglas Abrams & Rachel Carlton Abrams

The Science and Practice of Manual Therapy by Eyal Lederman

The Tao of Sexual Massage by Stephen Russell and Jurgen Kolb

The V Book: Vital Facts about the Vulva, Vestibule, Vagina and More by Dr. Elizabeth Stewart & Paula Spencer

Waking the Tiger: Healing Trauma by Peter A. Levine & Ann Frederick

My Journey as a Healer and Healing in Progress

> *"The secret of health for mind and body is not to mourn for the past, not to worry about the future, nor to anticipate troubles, but to live in the present moment wisely and earnestly."* BUDDHA

My journey as a healer has not been without its obstacles, for as I explained earlier my work has been met with as much opposition as it has support, but I continue to practice my healing for a number of reasons: firstly because I know it is my true calling in life; secondly because I have seen the remarkable results of my work; and thirdly because I categorically maintain that my work is needed and that no one else in the United Kingdom currently has the level of practical experience or the in-depth knowledge I have in the field of emotional detox and female ejaculation. It is certain that exploring many aspects of esoteric studies helps me to satisfy my thirsty brain but also gave me an insight into the areas in which my skill and passion lay.

Hundreds of heartfelt testimonials all give credit to my therapy methods and work as a healer. I continue be inspired by all of my clients and my learning journey as a healer continues. The stories of my clients are often traumatic, but their transformations are remarkable. I have so many accounts that I would love to share, but the bounds of client confidentiality prevent me, but here are some stories that I can share with you.

Transformations

Diana –

Today's client, Diana had discovered me through my website and had made her appointment with me in a moment of boldness. When she arrived for her first appointment she was very nervous, in fact she was so nervous that she was trembling with fear. Before the session began we just talked, we talked for over two hours. She told me her story of growing up in a commune in the UK, until the age of thirteen. She told me the harrowing account of how her own mother had sexually abused her since she was a toddler. Over the course of the abuse that she suffered from her mother she had experienced having things forcibly inserted into her yoni and was made to perform cunnilingus. Having suffered the ultimate betrayal from her mother, her father then began to sexually abuse and rape her. Eventually she fell pregnant as the result of being raped by her father.

Later in life as a teenager she has been subjected to a gang rape and one of the perpetrators had been considered a close friend. This woman's life had been subjected to a tyranny of abuse and betrayal.

Her story was one of abuse throughout the generations, with her grandfather having abused her mother and then this abuse was passed on in a crooked cycle. The abuse was passed off as rituals. Diana's brother had suffered the same abuse and indeed it was her brother's acknowledgement of his abuse and admission that he was going for therapy that had prompted her to come and see me.

She explained that both she and her brother had both had long periods of time when they had resigned themselves to thinking that they had imagined the abuse. They had both found the awful reality of their abuse unbearable and so took comfort in pretending it never happened.

Diana's brother has been in therapy for most of his life. Whilst Diana had been fortunate in finding a loving and supportive husband who was her rock. It was her husband who had chaperoned her to her first treatment session with me and who had given her the courage to keep the appointment.

There is no doubt as to the love that Diana and her spouse felt for each other, but she explained that when they made love she experienced no feelings in the yoni; she described feeling like a dead person. We spoke about the work that I did and she had knowledge of the yoni work, because she had once received yoni massage from another Sri Lankan healer, living in the UK and had felt some of the healing effects.

After speaking for a long while she had a shower and then we did breathing exercises, stretching and followed by a whole of body massage. She was relaxed, but there was no excitement and no pleasure gained from the experience. After the massage she said that she had enjoyed the massage and when I was doing the front massage she had no problems, then she explained that she had tension, in the back shoulders and neck.

She was quite open and then I did the yoni massage, but the yoni was tense and rigid. She had an hour concentrated yoni massage and she was very tense. We had a break and then she signalled that she wished to continue. I then spent a further hour and a half concentrating on yoni massage and eventually it became soft and surrendered and then I brought in the masculine energy and it was at this point that she felt pain and we stopped the treatment for a while, before resuming at her own pace. Each time we stopped and started again....the yoni was getting softer and less painful. This pattern continued and it was when she allowed me to work with her through the pain that she ejaculated.

Usually female ejaculation starts emotional release, but in Diana the emotions were supressed and so I warned her that she would feel the impact of emotional release in the next few days.

She was so happy after the session....she said that her yoni had never felt pleasure before and now she had some feeling. She didn't orgasm but ejaculated six times. This treatment did not yield climax, but a little pleasure was starting to be felt and this was a major breakthrough for her.

When the session was over she said that she was so happy that she had kept the appointment and said "that it's not even sexual" and instead it's the "most emotional of experiences". She couldn't cry and she told me, "I don't hug....I've never been hugged as a child," but after her session she did hug and she said "it felt like hugging a god". She said she couldn't believe that she could let go like that. She was amazed by the feeling of deep unconditional love that filled her during and after the treatment.

Her treatment sessions continue and slowly and gradually she is working through emotional detox.

Poppy –

When Poppy came to me she was scared of being alone for the rest of her life. Even though she was a qualified Brandon Bays journey therapist, she was struggling to resolve her inner turmoil and find a long lasting relationship.

Poppy's marriage had broken down, leaving her partner-less for 8yrs. She couldn't get a long term relationship even though she was actively looking. She was finding men, but they would just result in one night stands.

Poppy cannot remember any abuse, but she held shame in her system. As a child of 7 years or so, she was playing with a boy in the school toilet, and they came to explore each other's body. The boy went and told everyone in the class and she felt ashamed. She had held this shame for years. We did Deep Bodywork, yoni massage and ejaculation work and we talked about her desire to find long term love. Her sole purpose for coming for treatment was to find a special someone, but she didn't really believe it was possible.

When I was massaging her yoni Poppy started crying; she was releasing stored negative emotion. When I do the massage the clients sometimes see a video screen in their head, with past events being recalled in a very fast moving film and when she was seeing this, she saw the death of her infant brother and felt all the loss and sadness that was stored within her. She then released all the emotions connected with this event. In the yoni she was holding on to loss and shame. It is not just abuse that can be held in the yoni, but also anger, mistrust, shame, sadness, loss, bereavement and any other emotions.

She was hunting for a man, but they weren't chasing after her. Then after four sessions she suddenly had four men interested in her, she was spoilt for choice. After dating them all, she decided that one of them was special and that she wanted to settle down with him. He was a self-confessed womaniser who had a high flying job that allowed him to move from country to country and woman to woman. She liked him, but she feared that he would abandon her.

She continued sessions whilst seeing him and I gave her yoni exercises to practice and today they are still together and he is committed to her. Her Tantric Journey resulted in her finding and keeping the man of her dreams.

Josephine –

Josephine cannot remember whether she has been abused as a child or not, but she cannot trust men and this has impacted on her sex life, love life and relationships throughout her adult life. So when she came to see me she explained that her problem was that when she made love she couldn't orgasm, and if she masturbated she felt no pleasure. She wanted to experience an orgasm and during her first session with me she ejaculated and every consequent session she ejaculated, but the orgasm was elusive.

Ejaculation is about opening the Second Chakra, but orgasm is about opening all the Chakras and with Josephine we couldn't get past the solar plexus, because she had intimacy issues. So we decided to address her intimacy issues.

We established that Josephine gained pleasure from giving, but when it came to receiving she froze. She could not bypass this issue.

It was the fifth session that we challenged intimacy. After her ejaculation, I lay next to her in spoon position and immediately she evoked anger and sadness. Then I worked on the pressure points in the back of her neck "mouth of god". The more I massaged her, the more angry she got. Then she was given a pillow to beat and she then shouted and swore and got angry for fifteen minutes whilst she got her anger emotions out.

Then we continued with the massage and then after the massage she reproached me and said that I should not have challenged her intimacy without forewarning her and, I explained that I was trying to catch her off guard, because this is how we can begin to address the intimacy issues. It was a tough session.

So on the sixth session Josephine wanted some pleasure, so I focused on the yoni and she felt a little sensation and pleasure in the yoni, but there is much more work ahead of us and there are still many obstacles to overcome.

Now she has connected with her lifelong partner and comfortable with love, intimacy and her sexuality.

Sarah -

Sarah came to me because she couldn't have sex with her husband. She desperately wanted to be able to enjoy a full relationship with her husband and enjoy sexual pleasure.

She told me that from the age of six years old, her father would come into her room at night and sexually abuse her and that when her father left the room, very often her grandfather would come in and resume the abuse. As if this wasn't enough to bear, during the daytime her great grandfather would sexually abuse her and so three generations of her patriarchal family systematically abused her until she turned thirteen.

She had never felt any sense of orgasm or pleasure, but through regular Tantric Journey treatments she began to feel pleasure and achieved orgasm. Her husband recognised the change in her and he was curious and wanted to learn how to do my work. He came for sessions with her, but sadly he couldn't quite get the hang of the technique and his intentions turned out not be honourable as he wanted to use the technique with his many girlfriends not with his wife. Sarah and her husband eventually parted, but with her new found inner strength and having released her negative emotions, she was free to give and receive love.

Anna – (now a Tantric therapist herself)

Anna's father abused her as a child and when she was twenty years of age, she was diagnosed as having cervical cancer. She knew that she needed to find help and after looking on my website she decided to book a session. It was after her second session that she experienced emotional release. In her emotional state, she branded me a pervert and I didn't see her for a long period of time.

She went on to study holistic therapies and eventually came back to see me again after a couple of years, because she had started to realise the merit of my work through her studies. She became my client for two years and during this period she transformed.

When Anna first came to see me, she couldn't allow men near her and she had no chance of finding a partner. Today she is free from cancer, happily married and works as a Tantric Healer, treating men. This is an amazing transformation, but is typical of the type I see in clients every day.

Client Testimonials

Caroline Muir - Source School of Tantra - Maui, Hawaii, 26th June 2001

"Mal is a very kind and sensitive healer, utilising a marriage of his excellent massage skills, pure energy and loving kindness."

Francesca - London, 12th July 2001

"Mal's tantric training has helped me to relax and receive pleasure much more easily. I am now experiencing multiple orgasms with my boyfriend."

Dr Judy Kuriansky - New York, 25 January 2002

"Mal I cherish your friendship. What a joy you are to the world. A loving, giving soul with such a pure heart and healing and wise spirit. A gift indeed to all who know you."

Mrs Valerie - London, 5th February 2002

"Thank you for helping me see that there is no need to live in constant stress and for taking the time to show me a little bit of heaven." Valerie

Psychotherapist - Oakland, USA, 20th February 2002

"I strongly recommend Mal's sacred yoni massage for all women!"

Melanie - Therapist - Kingston, Surrey, 4th March 2002

"I was scared. I mean really scared... I also knew that I was not willing to live life as a non-sexual woman any more. Every day reminders that I can't enjoy sex like others can. Knowing that every relationship was doomed. I am half way through the treatment with Mal. At the beginning he said "Don't trust me - let me earn that trust," and he did. Only half way and I have discovered lust, pleasure and hope that I can enjoy a full sexual relationship. Mal does his job to the highest professional standards."

Lelani - Therapist - London, 1st October 2007

"I have had 6 sessions with Mal, and in every session we have been unpeeling the onion, and I have been challenged to let go of past barriers, bit for bit, in each session. Coming from a Christian background, my belief system was also challenged in quite a profound manner, and I have really had to maintain an open mind right throughout.

I have had irregular periods for over the past year and a half, as I was taking the contraceptive pill for several years since I was a teenager. My cycle was continuously over a 21 day period instead of 28, and I had gone for several acupuncture sessions to try and correct it, but it remained on 21 days. Since my treatment with Mal, my period has gone back to its natural cycle of 28 days.

Mal is an amazing healer, I cannot recommend him highly enough. Love, light and peace."

Kathleen - London, 6th December 2008

To have a healing session with Mal is to invite the darkness and shadows of your fear around your body and the feminine, sexual self, into the light. I knew when I heard of his work through Maya F, that his special Yoni Massage was something I wanted to experience. I think I was going through a period of "needing" to be seen by men and recognized as someone to love. Of course it wasn't happening, as the unspoken signal I was sending out, acted as a deterrent to the right kind of man. I felt pent-up and unsure of the "why's" surrounding it and seeing Mal was a lucid surrender.

I left a lot of things behind with the decision to see him and I knew even before the healing, that I wanted to experience the session completely. Before I arrived, though, I was feeling shy and even guilty around the idea. I was early for my appointment and he was still working, so I sat on the street corner by a tree and just looked at the sky and waited. Having these moments, gave me time to reflect on what it is I was seeking and why. When he sent a message saying I could come around, I was more relaxed and ready.

As we sat together cross-legged in his sanctuary with candles and music, a calm came over me and I knew that this man could hold me in a place that maybe no man ever had. He was so thorough and trusting and gentle. He asked me if I felt prepared to have the full

Yoni Massage and I knew this was the whole reason I was sitting before him--so without hesitating I said 'yes'. Truly, this was one of the greatest gifts to myself, to have asked for -- and to have received. There was never a moment of fear, angst or worry. He explained that he would first work with the whole of my body to do a healing massage and then into the realms of release.

The experience of being with a man who was not your partner, who was not a doctor and yet was working in a healing way with your body that was sensual, but not sexual, was a new kind of extraordinary. It was almost as if Mal was the true definition of a physical therapist for the feminine places we rarely permit ourselves to understand in our every day existence.

I felt held and safe... and completely honoured, in where he was taking me with his healing. With the Yoni Massage, it was as if he returned a part of me to myself. After the healing, I felt strong and pure, in a way. The urgent sense of needing to be seen or touched or kissed or adored by a man, seemed to dissipate. It has been three months and I am still in the feeling of how wondrous this healing was -- and I have been seeing a very sensuous man who loves and adores my body and person. I am the most relaxed I have ever been in a physical relationship. I am even surprising myself by the calm I have and the idea of "need" is no longer in my person.

The Yoni Massage with Mal was one of the most valuable reflections and experiences I have ever given myself. I have recommended him to those who are experiencing challenges with their partners or physical/sexual selves. Mal is tender, professional, guiding and kind and the journey he takes you on, is one to yourself. He does this with such integrity and honour. He leaves you with a sense that if you open and release your heart to the darkness of your fears, there is a place for you within it, that will reflect the joy that has been there all along.

My Love and Gratitude to You Mal,

Alvaro - Sri Lanka, 26th December 2008

It was quite a journey and I appreciate you coming and sharing your knowledge with me.

I look forward to learning more and exploring the world of Tantra. In that session I had to confront some deep seated fears and doubts that I thought I had dealt with. It really is deep and intense stuff and I believe you are doing a great service..

I hope that in time I learn more and work out my 90% and can assist in sharing the teachings with the world. First I am finding a reason why I want to do it. I have several but they need defining, I believe, in order to keep my focus and intent.

Ps. you are right after the fifth count during the "Yoni - Lingam" massage great things begin to happen to the woman... I manage to get to the end without fail on my part.

Janice - London, 16th February 2009

Dear Mal,

I saw you on Friday evening. Thank you so much for your wonderful knowledge.

I came to you at my lowest ebb. Your treatment was like receiving/experiencing a little bit of heaven. As the minutes moved on - the scales dropped off - I can vaguely see through the crack into the light.

I have had an intermittent headache over the weekend but also feel more grounded, less stressed, and optimistic.

I notice that you do 30 minute sessions of chanting with sounds. Toning is what you mentioned I needed as part of my process. Please may I make an appointment for a Friday or Monday whenever you can fit me in.

I also mentioned that I am a massage/psycho and hypno-therapist - and so as you can imagine - I am already thinking that I would like to move towards asking you to undertake to be my teacher and guide along the process - but all in the fullness of time, when you think I am ready. In the meantime I look forward to seeing you as much as I can afford. At the moment I don't even have a job - or a divorce!

If any of your students ever need a body to work on please may I volunteer? So all in all, many doors will now open. I look forward to the process.

Thank you again for your time, expertise, patience, and kindness. Hugs and love.

Susan - London, 1ˢᵗ March 2009

Dear Mal,

Thank you for a wonderful experience of Tantra on Friday. I haven't had any negative reactions - at least so far! I was very tired on Friday evening and slept well. I'll write a proper testimonial in a few days and send it to you. In the meantime, I wanted you to know that I found it both an interesting and enjoyable experience.

I'll make another appointment sometime in April, when I return from Canada.

With Best Wishes, Susan.

Helen - Freelance Journalist - London, 16th January 2010

Hi Mal,

Thank you. It really is remarkable how your treatment is working. I had been dubious at the start when you told me that you would win my trust but you certainly have and have given me great strength during this tough patch.

I have found the advice you have given me extremely insightful and calming and can feel myself growing stronger through it. At the moment I feel I am on something of a precipice between feeling despair and letting go of all fear and embracing a deeper sense of happiness and resilience. It feels like a battle with the mind that, once won, will probably never need to be fought again. I definitely think this is giving me a real sense of how your treatment works that I will be able to explain and pass on with conviction.

Regarding the massage therapy work, I feel I have been holding myself back for the past year, getting some positive responses but lacking the courage to throw myself into it. Perhaps it is as you say that I am seeking to become more open by working as a therapist but have not been ready to open myself up until now so have hindered my own progress. I would love to become an excellent massage therapist and am so grateful you have offered to coach me in that.

I'm looking forward to seeing you on Monday. Hope you're having a nice weekend.

Love, Helen.

Torik & Roxie - London, October 2011

Hi Mal,

First of all, can I just say thanks so much again for that wonderful evening. I was left breathless, excited, amazed, and ultimately extremely fulfilled.

Unfortunately I haven't had a chance to practise anymore just yet. I was hoping to try it over the last weekend, but I still had a problem with my leg, which worsened on Saturday night. Hopefully with all being well, I aim to do it in the next few days.

Despite that however, I would like to explain the effect that it has had on me.

The whole process from start to finish was one of the most, if not THE most beautiful and heart-warming experiences I have ever had.

I really enjoyed your thorough and heart felt explanation before we carried out any body work, you made everything so clear, very simple to understand, leaving me feeling comfortable and at ease. And one of the most important things to note, and as you explained very well, that only a small amount of it was about the technique, but the rest was about love and intention.

During the time we worked on the body and the time since then, it has uncovered a lot of areas that I didn't even know existed. It was such a fulfilling experience; the massages were soft and tender, the breath work was deep and controlled and the ejaculation was simple and very loving.

I realise now how importantitis to practise this, because fundamentally I believe it has the ability to heal a wide variety of different issues, and can make relationships far more exciting, truthful and ultimately brings couples even closer together.

This is certainly what it has done for me, and as the time has passed since the last session with yourself, it has already had a massively positive impact for me and Roxie. I can't wait to practise it again, and as you so clearly explained it doesn't even matter about the outcome, but my truth and intention has never been more present for me than it is now, and that is in very large part to the way you brought this to us.

It has made me feel more confident and relaxed about myself and about my relationship, but at the same time also very excited and energized. The beauty and essence about the whole thing is that it is so very natural, and as such, it has touched me in quite a profound way, and ultimately left me feeling even more loving, and a deeper love that goes beyond anything I have experienced before in a relationship.

I cannot recommend this enough, and I will encourage as many people as I can to experience this at least once if not several times in their life.

Thanks again for showing me the way. With loving regards,

Aphrodite - Therapist - London, October 2011

I have always enjoyed giving massage and making people feel relaxed....then I discovered Tantra. I had read a lot about it and never knew what all the hype was all about until receiving a beautiful Tantric Massage from Mal.

Having been brought up in a strict upbringing where sexuality is viewed in a negative way, my experience of sexuality was supressed. Mal helped me to work on my Chakras - especially my Heart

Chakra - the ability to love freely without fear or self-consciousness, and my Crown chakra to help with fear and depression.

KTA - London, 7th October 2011

Hello Mal,

I am back in my job here in the Bank Colombia. I have been here for 3 weeks and it has been difficult to adapt again, because I really enjoyed my 6 months there. Today, I have to tell you THANK U, because London hadn't been same without you. You made better and more comfortable my stay in London.

I have missed you a lot and I have been remembering you all the time...

Eyeryday I wake up and I say: "THANKS GOD, BECAUSE THESE WERE THE BEST MONTHS IN MY LIFE. THANK YOU FOR THE ANGELS THAT YOU PUT IN MY WAY, I WILL ALWAYS REMEMBER MY DAYS IN LONDON AND THESE BEAUTIFUL PEOPLE THAT GAVE ME A HAND."

You were one of these angels for me...

I recognize that I love my family and I missed them a lot, that my city is beautiful, that we have the best weather in the world, that people here is very warm and we have everything we need to live well and loved...but now, I must accept that I don't have any barriers, that there are many possibilities in the world and I can do whatever I want... For that reason I know that we can see us again and there are no limits to find us and to hug us again.

THANK U, GRACIAS, GRATZIE, OBRIGADO!

Kisses,

Jennie - Coach, Empathy, Writer - **London, 14ᵗʰ October 2011**

Embarking on a Tantric Healing Journey takes courage. Your healer needs to be a master in their field and also to be kind, caring and infinitely patient. Mal has these qualities in abundance. I am really grateful to Mal for his help and guidance in helping me let go of some long held blocks.

Leila - London, March 2012

Like anyone else, every year of my adult life I have started with pockets full of various 'new year resolutions'. Every year I promise to be a better person, work harder, be more focused, love and cherish life.

But at some point of the year I manage to dump all my 'resolutions' and go back to square one- where I become myself again - a semi-depressed mother with an obscure mind and lack of serenity. Oh, don't get me wrong! I love my child and adore my partner, it is just a feeling of gap that needs to be filled in my brain or heart or some might call it a soul. I tried so many things and never managed to find peace, and this time once again I am making a resolution to find peace through Tantra. I am giving myself a year to see a change, and will be posting my reflections right here.

Why Tantra? Saying frankly, I don't know. After trying studying and practicing various philosophies that seemed to shape my current "I" (but failed to bring the expected change), I returned back to a very special person who offered his help many years ago. Back then I rejected his offer, and 8 years on, full of hope I found him again. I guess the saying "When the student is ready the master appears" suits my case well.

I always had interest in Eastern philosophies. Through my late teenagehood I was obsessed with Osho's teachings, whose spiritual path combined elements Hinduism, Buddhism, Taoism, Christianity and many other religious and philosophic traditions, humanistic psychology and meditation; then I embraced Islamic philosophy and practice and here I am...in search once again...

Back to "the master" thing; I met Mal in 2003. He is the pioneer Tantric therapist in London. We talked about my interest in Eastern philosophies, my constant search for love and satisfaction and inability to find it. He then suggested to study (or perhaps explore) Tantra. I was open minded and excited, but after my first session, I felt overwhelmed and couldn't cope with the tsunami of various emotions and instead of returning back to Mal, I had suppressed my emotions for many more years. I decided to see Mal again for his advice 8 years later. This time; I was clear about my questions and my needs and was ready for a long journey to reach my goal. In fact- my ultimate goal- to achieve serenity and love.

Sooooo, I was offered a journey - Tantric Journey, that promises to bring the healing, and I am up for it. I will be seeing my 'master' 3 times a month, which makes about 40 times a year. I will posting my reflections of every single training session and perhaps additional postings of my own mini researches on Tantric life.

I guess that is it... So long!

Gabrielle - Naturopath - London, January 2013

Hello Mal,

It's nearly a week since my session; the results are still developing beautifully. After a few days of feeling and looking a bit pale and low in energy, today I had a client for Bodywork; the quality of my work seems positively affected, I had a really good time too! My family relationships are nicer; I am less edgy and gentler, although firm. My energy is better...even my body odours are improved!

I'm experiencing my body more as I used to in the Sannyas Commune

- as one flowing gorgeous organism, open, with immediate potential for pleasure and swift release of trauma.

Your brochure is a professional piece of work, and I have no hesitation in handing it around to the right people.

PR - London, March 2013

Mal is working with me on some very challenging material which dates from my upbringing to secure a man or else be a nobody, an oddity.

He has the skill and the courage to gain my trust, even though I have betrayed my own truth over and over again in intimate relations with men.

This deep body- work is beginning to relax and melt the longstanding numbness, frigidity and physical pain. My husband and I are able to relate again, and the mysterious enmity that has separated us is releasing and bringing in so much tenderness and love.

I thank Mal for this, with all my heart.

Anna - Vienna, 31st March 2013

Dear Mal,

I have arrived back in my home in Vienna. And enjoying a very quiet and laid back Easter Sunday. Yesterday my heart was overflowing with Love and I send you telepathic message full of thankfulness and kindness. You are a great man that is there for the women to heal and find trust in the men (again). I am so glad you exist :)

I have recommended you to all female friends I have met since meeting you. Looking forward to hearing from you and seeing you again.

Virginia - London, 30ᵗʰ March 2013

Dear Mal,

Easter in Spanish is "Pascuas" which means Path. It reminds us of the path from Slavery to Freedom. The Path from Death to Life. Very symbolic. Because I worked so much to break free and I'm still working, I don't want to miss the chance to thank you (someone once told me that chances are so few and life's so short ...) as you were part of it.

A good time for insight these days. At least for me; and also for gratitude. You've helped me so much. Thanks again.

For everything mentioned above and because I really feel I like the woman I've become, I wanted to share it with you.

Thanks Dear Friend! Happy Easter!

Risako - London, 8ᵗʰ May 2013

Hi Mal,

Thanks for giving me the wonderful session yesterday. I've arrived at Paris today.

It's been great experience, and I feel wonderful! I feel I've shed a skin. I hope the boxes you opened for me don't close too quickly. It is such an exciting feeling that I am moving forward positively. Without your help, I would not experience like this.

Thanks again, and I hope to see you soon!! Lots of love,

Nueng - Chang Mai - Thailand, 10th August 2013

Hi Mal,

I'm fine here in Bangkok and feel so grateful to know you and receive the treatment from you. It's truly special. I've never had that feeling or experience in my life like that before. It's very intimate and healing way of treatment. You really broke me open in some way (in a good way).. I can't explain it, but I feel it. One thing I feel is like I got a feeling of being proud to be a woman again... Thank you for a sincere love and relationship you gave to me, it's really special. And yes you got magic hands Mal.

I'd be pleased to meet you again when you are in Thailand... just let me know.

Have a safe trip back home... Love & Light

Catherine Oxenberg - London, 20th Nov 2013

I have been working with Mal since January 2013.

Mal is a very skilled healer, and my marriage has benefited a lot from his guidance. I have recommended him too many of my friends & family.

Dakini Sophie - London, 19th Oct 2014

Wow, my body instantly recognised that Mal is a very learned and experienced practitioner. It was so easy to surrender to his powerful Bodywork and gentle manner. I had lots of emotional release happening, it was a profound experience. I plan to go back for more as I've felt better than ever generally and much more open to pleasure since our first session.

Stacy Burgess - London, 1st Nov 2014

Mal is very professional and experienced person, I have ever met. He has healing ability on very higher level. His understanding of individual's needs and emotions are on higher level and healing is very powerful. As soon as Mal touches my body, he knows where is exactly the imbalance and the way he handles gentle soothing way you like to completely surrender to him. He is just amazing and the best therapist to be a Tantric healer. He has released all my emotional blockages and I am a completely new person by the time he finishes his journey. I am Mal's regular client and love to recommend him to others.

Glossary of Terms

Amrita:

"Referred to as Devine Nectar or the drink of the gods, which grants women immortality. This flows from two locations:

1. Amrita is a fluid that can flow from the pituitary gland down the throat in deep states of meditation (Third Eye Chakra Opening)
2. This Divine Nectar - cups of warm clear liquid gushing or spraying out of the female's genital area. Once a woman's "channels" are open she can easily release her sacred waters through self-pleasuring. Her time alone becomes not only fun and pleasurable, but gives her direct connection to her own divinity, her own power, to the goddess within her essence. She might "offer" this gift of liquid energy to her loved ones or to her own personal belief of what spirit is to her. It is alleged to be sweet-tasting. Currently in the West, this is known as Female Ejaculation or Squirting (Second Chakra Opening)"
                                                                    - Wikipedia

Chakra:

An energy centre in the subtle body along the spinal axis through which consciousness manifests in human form; lit., a spinning wheel. There are seven major Chakras in the body which are now known to

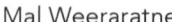

be in parallel locations to our hormone producing glands, endocrine system

Kama:

Desire; an intrinsic aspect of divine will; the first step of the descent of consciousness toward manifestation of the material world

Lingam:

A Sanskrit term of reverence for the statues and images of the god Shiva's genital organ; lingam is also used as a technical term for the male penis

Yoni:

Vagina or female genitals. It's the symbol of the Goddess Shakti, consort of God Shiva

Prana:

Life force, the vital force that nourishes both body and mind; the breath of life; five major aspects are prana, apana, vyana, udana, and samana; and five minor aspects: naga, kurma, krikara, devadatta, and dhananjaya; also the cosmic vibratory power underlying creation

Kundalini:

"Coiled up energy"; the dormant potential energy in all living beings; self-contained totally independent locus point; a point of reference which is saturated with the principle of creativity

9 781504 994156